Pharmacology

Pharmacology

Robert S. Sloviter, PhD

Assistant Professor of Pharmacology and Neurology
Columbia University College of Physicians and Surgeons
New York, New York

CREOG

Basic Science Monograph in Obstetrics and Gynecology

Council on Resident Education in Obstetrics and Gynecology
600 Maryland Avenue SW, Washington DC 20024

Library of Congress Cataloging in Publication Data
Main entry under title:

Pharmacology.

(CREOG basic science monograph in obstetrics and gynecology)
Prepared under the direction of the Committee on Education and Curriculum of the Council on Resident Education in Obstetrics and Gynecology, with the assistance of Robert S. Sloviter.
Includes bibliographical references.
1. Pharmacology.   I. Sloviter, Robert S., 1950-
II. Council on Resident Education in Obstetrics and Gynecology. Committee on Education and Curriculum.   III. Series.
[DNLM: 1. Pharmacology. QV 4 P53605]
PM300.P517 1984   615′.7   83-24076
ISBN 0-915473-00-3
  3 4 5 / 8

**The development of this Basic Science Monograph
in Pharmacology was made possible by a grant from
Parke-Davis.**

Contents

Preface

Modern medical practice is characterized by the degree to which it is based on scientific fact. Practice by intuition or anecdotal experiences, which may have been laudable at one point in medical history, is now condemned because it cannot withstand, or is not subjected to, the scrutiny of "scientific method." Therefore, the quality of a physician's practice is greatly influenced by the extent of the individual's scientific knowledge.

Medical education reflects a marked heterogeneity—in both the academic setting of medical school and the clinical orientation of residency programs. Today's rapid pace of scientific discoveries has an impact on the practice of obstetrics and gynecology. This fact dictates the continuing identification of basic science information most pertinent to the specialty.

In response to this need, the Council on Resident Education in Obstetrics and Gynecology (CREOG), under the direction of the CREOG Committee on Education and Curriculum, has developed a series of basic science monographs. These monographs are designed to review principles related to, but not necessarily clinically correlated with, direct patient care. The information in this series has been carefully selected to form a foundation for the application of basic science principles in a clinical environment. Such a background is an essential part of postgraduate education—both in residency and in continuing medical education.

Intentionally, the monographs are neither all encompassing nor exhaustively detailed; textbooks and other reference sources are available for more in-depth study. Rather, the review of basic science as reflected in this monograph series serves as a basis for discussion, amplification, and exploration of information particularly relevant to reproductive health. The content will be reviewed periodically and, based on critiques and feedback received, revised to ensure currency and applicability to the specialty.

To enhance the authoritativeness and usefulness of the monographs, specialists well versed in their respective fields were invited to serve as authors. CREOG is indebted to Robert Sloviter, PhD, for writing the text of this monograph on *Pharmacology*, which in eight chapters, outlined and indexed in detail, provides an overview of pharmacologic principles and mechanisms that are particularly relevant to obstetrics and gynecology.

1

General Principles of Drug Action

The primary goal of pharmacologic therapy is to deliver a drug molecule to its site of action (its receptor) at a concentration that can produce the desired biologic response. Delivery of a drug to its receptor for the desired effect involves its absorption and distribution; the subsequent removal of the drug from its site of action involves its metabolism and excretion. Every drug molecule has its own "fingerprint," a unique combination of molecular weight, size, three-dimensional shape, lipid/water solubility, acid/base characteristics, susceptibility to chemical transformation, and similarity in structure to endogenous substances. These properties determine a drug's relative ability to be absorbed and distributed to the site of action, the nature of the interaction with its receptor, and its tendency to be transformed and eliminated.

ABSORPTION

Movement of Molecules Across Membranes

The absorption into the body of any drug, regardless of the route of administration, can be regarded in terms of movement across biologic barriers that separate the drug molecule from its receptor site.

PASSIVE DIFFUSION

Most compounds are absorbed through the gut wall, the skin, or mucous membranes by passive diffusion, a process that does not involve the expenditure of cellular energy or the active involvement of biologic transport processes. There are three main types of passive diffusion.

Filtration of Small Molecules. Since most capillary beds have gaps between the endothelial cells, small molecules can cross these barriers by simple filtration. This involves the bulk flow of the aqueous solvent and the small molecules dissolved in it. This process takes place in the small intestine, where the relatively small

3

intercellular gaps (4 nm) permit filtration of small molecules, and in the capillaries, where the larger gaps (40 nm) permit filtration of larger molecules.

Lipid-Soluble Drugs. In the passive diffusion of nonionizable drugs through lipid membranes, the rate of membrane passage is proportional to the relative lipid/water solubility of the drug and the concentration gradient across the membrane. The more lipid-soluble the drug, the more readily it dissolves in, and therefore crosses, the membrane.

Ionizable Compounds. Ionizable molecules (weak acids and bases) form an equilibrium between the charged and uncharged forms of the same molecule, depending on the pH of the solvent in which they are dissolved. For a weak acid, the presence of a high concentration of hydrogen ions in the surrounding solvent shifts the equilibrium in the direction of the un-ionized state. Hence, at a low pH, the weak acid aspirin is predominantly uncharged (protonated) and more readily crosses the stomach wall and enters the blood. At a high pH, the aspirin molecules are predominantly in the charged (unprotonated) form and are less readily absorbed from the stomach. The reverse is true for weak bases. At a low pH (high hydrogen ion concentration), the nitrogen molecule of many weak bases accepts a proton, becoming charged (NH_3^+); at a high pH (low hydrogen ion concentration), however, the nitrogen molecule donates its proton to the solvent and reverts to the uncharged state (NH_2). Since uncharged molecules cross lipid membranes more easily than do their charged counterparts, the pH of the solution in which an ionizable drug is dissolved greatly affects the ability of the drug to cross a membrane. This principle also applies to the distribution of an ionizable drug into and out of body fluids of different pH (eg, blood/urine).

CARRIER-MEDIATED TRANSPORT

Many drug molecules are too large to be filtered through intercellular gaps or membrane pores or are too highly charged to diffuse passively through lipid membranes. These compounds can cross membranes via biologic carrier mechanisms that cells normally use to transport endogenous molecules. Some of these carriers require no expenditure of cellular energy (facilitated diffusion), while others do require energy (active transport).

Facilitated Diffusion. In passive diffusion, the rate of movement is determined largely by the concentration gradient across the membrane; as the concentration of the molecule increases on one side of the membrane, there is a proportional increase in the rate of diffusion across the membrane. In the case of facilitated diffusion, the transport of a molecule depends on the availability of a membrane-bound carrier substance that, together with the drug concentration, determines the rate of passage. Until the carrier substance is saturated with the molecule to be transported, an increase in the substrate concentration increases the rate of drug transport. The presence of other molecules that can be transported via the same carrier can block the rate of drug entry, however. Therefore, these carrier-mediated processes are saturable, concentration-dependent, and competitive transport systems. The biologic development of these carriers allows the selective entry of desired molecules through normally impenetrable barriers. In this sense, pharmacologic intervention often involves "tricking" a carrier into accepting a substrate (the drug) that, although foreign, is similar in structure to one required by the cell.

Active Transport. In contrast to diffusion, in which drug molecules move across membranes as a result of a concentration gradient, active transport involves the use of energy in order to move solutes against a concentration gradient. For example, because the concentration of sodium ions in extracellular fluid is higher than that in intracellular fluid, sodium ions tend to move into the cell down their concentration gradient. This is undesirable in most cases, since the ability of cells to exclude sodium is necessary for the maintenance of charge separation across the membrane. Therefore, the cell membrane is relatively impermeable to sodium ions, and a transport mechanism (Na^+-K^+ adenosinetriphosphatase [ATPase]) works actively to exclude sodium ions against a concentration gradient. Similarly, some cells need to sequester substances intracellularly, and these cells must use an energy-requiring active transport process to force entry of these required molecules against a concentration gradient favoring exit.

Factors Affecting Absorption

DISSOLUTION

In order to be absorbed, a drug must first be in solution. Therefore, the rate of absorption is affected by the rate of dissolution of a tablet, for example. This factor can be used to provide rapid delivery of a drug (a solid dosage form designed to dissolve rapidly) or to provide a slow supply of drug (coated tablets). A similar situation exists for drugs suspended or dissolved in an oil or wax depot preparation. Because the only drug available to cross a membrane is the drug that is in solution and comes in contact with the absorbing membrane, the rate at which a drug is liberated from a solid dosage form or from an intramuscular or subcutaneous depot form can be either an obstacle to rapid absorption or a means to provide long-duration delivery.

ROUTES OF ADMINISTRATION

In addition to the chemical interaction between a solute and the membrane, a large number of variables contribute to the rate of absorption in vivo. Also of great importance are the amount of membrane surface area available to the drug and the rate of blood flow on the inner surface of the membrane that removes absorbed drug from one side, thereby affecting the concentration gradient. These factors can be used to advantage, depending on whether the drug administered is given for its local effects or its systemic effects.

Gastrointestinal Tract

Sublingual Administration. The thin epithelial lining of the mouth and the high rate of blood flow through the tissues of the mouth permit rapid absorption of some drugs. The small surface area available to the drug and the problem of patient compliance preclude the routine use of this route of administration, however. The sublingual route of administration is commonly used for angina pectoris when the relief of pain must be rapid and the drug of choice (nitroglycerin) would be metabolized by the liver after intestinal absorption.

Stomach and Small Intestine. The stomach has a very small absorptive surface area compared with that of the small intestine. The stomach lining is relatively smooth, whereas the small intestine mucosa consists of villi and microvilli that expand the available surface area enormously. The stomach and small intestine also differ in the pH of their contents. The stomach contents are acidic; those of the small intestine are more alkaline. Because the absorption rate of lipid-soluble drugs is independent of pH, their rate of absorption is greater in the small intestine than in the stomach, owing to the greater absorptive area of the intestine. For the weak acid or base, however, both the absorptive area and the pH must be considered.

As mentioned earlier, the weak acid aspirin is protonated and therefore predominantly in the uncharged form at an acidic pH. Since uncharged molecules can be readily absorbed, aspirin is rapidly absorbed from the stomach. In the more alkaline pH of the small intestine, the aspirin is predominantly in the unprotonated form, ie, the charged form of a weak acid. Therefore, if two identical doses of aspirin in two identical volumes of water are placed simultaneously in the lumen of the empty stomach and in the lumen of the empty small intestine, consideration of the pH effects on ionized and un-ionized forms of the drug suggests that the drug is absorbed more rapidly from the stomach. This is incorrect. The small intestine provides such an enormous absorptive surface area that, even though less aspirin is in the uncharged form, the small uncharged amount is very rapidly absorbed. Instantly, as the uncharged form of the drug disappears from the intestinal lumen, the equilibrium between charged and uncharged forms reestablishes itself, providing more of the uncharged form to be absorbed. Absorption from the stomach is greater than that from the small intestine only if expressed per unit of absorptive surface area.

Large Intestine. The remainder of a drug that was partially absorbed from the stomach and small intestine can be absorbed from the large intestine. Although lacking microvilli, the absorptive surface of the large intestine is considerable. Rectal administration of drugs is convenient when a patient is unconscious or when unpleasant-tasting drugs must be used. In addition, the blood flow from the lower portion of the rectum bypasses the liver, and the drug absorbed by the rectal route is not subjected to a first-pass effect. This is an important consideration for any drug that is rapidly metabolized by the liver.

Parenteral Routes

Intravenous Administration. For systemic distribution of drugs, administration of drug into the blood is obviously the most direct route. Intravenous (IV) administration makes it possible to administer a known dose rapidly, which is, of course, useful in emergencies. It also circumvents the gastrointestinal (GI) tract when a drug is unpleasant-tasting, poorly absorbed, or irritating to other tissues. In addition, circumventing gastric absorption avoids early metabolism of the drug by the liver. However, the IV route requires precautions, such as sterile procedures. Furthermore, unlike a drug that has been administered orally, a drug that has been administered intravenously cannot be removed. Rapid IV injection of any drug with respiratory depressant activity (eg, morphine, heroin, or barbiturate) can deliver to the brain such a high concentration of the drug that breathing ceases. When given orally or slowly by the IV route, the same dose would not reach the same high concentration in the brain and would, therefore, not be lethal. IV injection can also be given inadvertently when subcutaneous, intramuscular, or epidural injection is attempted. This requires caution, especially when the drug being administered has known cardiopulmonary or CNS effects.

Intramuscular and Subcutaneous Injection. With the intramuscular (IM) and subcutaneous routes of administration, a drug is injected directly into tissue; the only barrier between the drug and the blood is the capillary cell. The main determinants of the rate at which the drug is absorbed into the blood are the rate of blood flow through the injected area and the amount of capillary surface area available to the drug for absorption. One way to affect the rate of absorption is to alter the blood flow through the area. During rest, the rate of absorption is similar after either IM or subcutaneous injection. The rate of IM absorption can be increased by exercise, however, since the rate of skeletal muscle blood flow is increased by sympathetic activation of arteriolar β-adrenergic receptors during exercise. Conversely, decreasing the rate of local blood flow by injecting a vasoconstrictor decreases the rate of absorption from the site of injection. This is commonly used in dentistry when epinephrine is injected with a local anesthetic. The α-adrenergic receptor agonist activity of epinephrine (it possesses both α- and β-adrenergic receptor agonist activity) constricts the local blood vessels, thus keeping the anesthetic in the tissue for a longer period of time.

The rate of drug absorption from the injection site can be increased by increasing the area of absorptive surface available to a subcutaneously injected drug. This can be done by subcutaneous injection of hyaluronidase, an enzyme that digests the subcutaneous connective tissue and thus permits the bolus injection to spread for a greater distance under the skin. Another way to increase the absorptive surface area is to give the same total dose in the same total volume, but to give it in several small-volume injections, thereby increasing the surface area in contact with the drug. For drugs that are not irritating and that cannot be given by mouth, the subcutaneous and IM routes of administration are not only safer than IV injections, but also avoid early metabolism of the drug by the liver.

Pulmonary Absorption. Volatile gases, such as anesthetics, and rapidly metabolized drugs can be administered in a mist. The thin membranes of the lung and the enormous surface area available for absorption make the pulmonary route of administration effective. Like the IV, subcutaneous, IM, sublingual, and rectal routes, the pulmonary route also avoids early hepatic metabolization of the administered drug.

Epidural Injection. Used in obstetric practice for the purpose of blocking nerve conduction in the sensory nerves innervating the pelvic area, the epidural route of administration involves the injection of local anesthetic into the tissue near the dura mater, which forms a protective sheath around the spinal cord. The drug diffuses passively through the dura, into the CSF, and into the spinal cord and nerves. The drug effect is terminated by the diffusion of the drug into the blood and surrounding tissue and by metabolism of the drug by tissue enzymes. The main hazards of this route of administration are the possible leakage of CSF if the dura is inadvertently punctured and the possible injection of anesthetic directly into blood vessels in the region. Therefore, during slow injection of local anesthetic, the possible adverse effects of IV drug injection, such as CNS excitation, must be kept in mind.

Intrathecal Injection. The intrathecal route of administration involves the injection of local anesthetic directly into the fluid surrounding the spinal nerves that transmit pelvic sensations to the brain. The processes that terminate drug action are the same as those for the epidural route. Since puncture of the dura is required for intrathecal injection, the possible leakage of CSF and subsequent neurologic symptoms (eg, headache, nausea, or dizziness) must be considered.

Other Routes of Administration. Drugs can be delivered to a specific region for a local effect by many other routes. These include topical, intracardiac, intraperitoneal, intrauterine, and intraarticular injection. Their uses are restricted, but the principles described earlier also apply to these routes.

DISTRIBUTION

The distribution of a drug describes the movement of the drug throughout the body after it has been absorbed into the body. To get to its site of action, a drug may traverse the capillary wall into the extracellular water and then cross the cellular membrane into the intracellular water. A drug that can cross all barriers is said to be dissolved in the total body water. This does not always occur, however.

Volume of Distribution

The way in which the body handles a particular drug can partially be described by the "volume of distribution." If a large molecule that cannot leave the bloodstream is injected into the bloodstream, the total volume into which it can distribute is the volume of the blood. Therefore, its volume of distribution is said to be approximately 3 liters, the volume of plasma in a 70-kg person. If a drug crosses the capillary wall into the extracellular water, but does not enter the cells of the body, its volume of distribution is the volume of extracellular water. If a small, lipid-soluble drug has been injected, its volume of distribution may be the entire volume of body water, approximately 40 liters.

The volume of distribution should not be taken too literally. If the blood is sampled and the drug measured after the IV injection of 1 mg of a drug that is very actively accumulated in a particular organ, the plasma concentration may be extremely low, perhaps 1 ng/ml. The volume of distribution is calculated by dividing the total amount of drug in the body by the concentration of the drug in plasma (usually extrapolated from a plasma decay curve). In this case, the volume of distribution is 1000 liters despite the fact that the total body water is only 40 liters and the person could displace 70 liters at most. Therefore, the volume of distribution should not be viewed as the volume of a specific tissue, organ, or "compartment," but as an indication of the drug's distribution in the many different compartments (both fluid and organ compartments) of the body. If a drug is highly bound by plasma proteins, for example, a large proportion of the drug may remain in the blood, and the drug is said to have a relatively small volume of distribution. This does not mean, however, that the small fraction of drug that does leave the blood is incapable of distributing widely throughout the body.

Factors Affecting Distribution

SIZE, LIPID SOLUBILITY, AND IONIZATION

All the chemical characteristics of a drug that affect its absorption also affect its distribution, since both processes can be viewed as movements across biologic barriers. Therefore, lipid-soluble drugs, which cross most barriers passively without regard for membrane pores, intercellular gaps, or uptake mechanisms, often distribute throughout the body. Similarly, small molecules generally gain wide access to most body compartments.

More complicated is the distribution of weak acids and bases. For these compounds, it may be helpful to view the body in terms of "pH zones." According to this view, the blood and extracellular water have a pH of 7.4; the milk, a pH of 7.0; the stomach, a pH of 2.0; and the small intestine, a pH of 0.8. The urine pH can be changed at will by administering a weak acid or base. When introduced into the blood, a weak acid or base distributes to all compartments differently and forms an equilibrium in each compartment between the charged and uncharged forms of the drug. Since milk is more acidic than blood, more of the weak base amphetamine that diffuses into the milk is charged than is the amphetamine in the blood. The charged amphetamine does not diffuse back passively; therefore, the concentration of amphetamine is higher in the milk than in the blood. At a urine pH of 8.0, more of the amphetamine in the urine is uncharged and, therefore, diffusible back into the blood. When an equilibrium is reached, the concentration in the urine is lower than in the blood. After a large ingestion of amphetamine, it is desirable to increase its rate of excretion by acidification of the urine with ammonium chloride. The amphetamine that goes from blood to urine by glomerular filtration becomes predominantly charged at an acid pH, is trapped in the urine, and is excreted. Clearly, an understanding of zonal pH and the acid/base characteristics of a drug makes it possible to deduce where in the body a drug is in low concentration, where it is in high concentration, and how its rate of elimination from the body may be affected to advantage.

BLOOD FLOW

After IV injection, a drug reaches relatively high concentrations quickly in tissues with a high blood flow rate. This is the initial phase of drug distribution. For example, the highly lipid-soluble anesthetic thiopental produces anesthesia within seconds after IV injection because the brain is mostly lipid and because the rate of blood flow to the brain, kidney, and heart is high compared with that to muscle, fat, skin, bone, and intestine. Shortly after administration, however, the thiopental distributes more completely, and an equilibrium forms between each tissue of the body and the blood. Since thiopental is highly lipid-soluble, the body fat is a site of loss, causing a rapid decrease in brain concentration and, as a result, consciousness. Thus, thiopental induces surgical anesthesia quickly, but for only a short time.

PLASMA PROTEIN BINDING

Drugs are useful because they interact chemically with a biologic receptor and, by doing so, cause a biologic response. The chemical properties of drugs also result in two types of unwanted interaction. One is the interaction between the drug and a receptor that mediates a biologic response that is not the primary intention of the therapy. For example, a muscarinic cholinergic receptor antagonist used to treat parkinsonism (desired effect) also causes a dry mouth (undesired effect) by acting on acetylcholine receptors in the salivary gland. The other type of undesired drug interaction is between the drug and a body constituent that does not mediate a biologic response. The circulating plasma proteins to which many drugs bind can be viewed as a major site of loss or, conversely, as a depot for many drugs.

Three concepts about plasma protein binding are particularly important:

1. There is a chemical equilibrium between the proportion of drug in the plasma that is bound to plasma proteins and that which is free. Each drug has its own bound/free ratio, depending on the nature of its chemical interaction with the protein.

2. Only free drug exerts a pharmacologic effect or distributes from the blood to other tissues or fluids of the body. As free drug leaves the blood, the bound/free equilibrium is instantly reestablished by a net release of some of the bound drug by the plasma protein.

3. Many drugs bind to the same protein sites; therefore, one drug can displace another, resulting in an abrupt and potentially dangerous increase in free drug concentration.

Protein binding can greatly affect the distribution of a drug. In starvation or liver disease, in which there is a decrease in plasma proteins, an "average" dose of a protein-bound drug could be an overdose.

For some drugs, plasma proteins act as a drug depot or reservoir. A highly bound drug is released from plasma proteins at a rate proportional to its metabolism or excretion. If a drug must be present in the body for a long time to produce its desired effect (eg, an antibiotic), the administration of a highly bound drug maintains a therapeutic concentration for longer than does the administration of an unbound drug. Furthermore, if the bound drug is released only at low plasma drug concentrations, the free drug available to produce a biologic effect may be below the necessary therapeutic concentration. In this case, the plasma proteins are regarded as a site of loss, rather than as a depot or reservoir.

TISSUE BINDING

Just as plasma proteins can bind drugs and affect their distribution, so can other tissues of the body. The antimalarial compound chloroquine, for example, binds avidly to DNA and is found in the liver, spleen, lung, and kidney at 200 to 700 times the plasma concentration. Therefore, these tissue binding sites must be saturated with a large primary dose if therapeutic plasma concentrations of chloroquine are to be reached. Other tissues also act as reservoirs or sites of loss. Tetracyclines and heavy metals bind to bone, and the total body fat can be viewed as a "deep compartment" for many lipid-soluble drugs and fat-soluble vitamins. If the return of a drug from a deep compartment into the blood maintains a therapeutic plasma drug concentration, the tissue is regarded as a reservoir. If the drug is returned in a concentration too low to produce a biologic response, the tissue is regarded as a site of loss.

BLOOD-BRAIN BARRIER

An understanding of the blood-brain barrier begins with an understanding of the reason for its existence. The brain and spinal cord function normally only when the ionic and chemical composition of the extracellular fluid is held within very narrow limits of normality. Neurotransmitters mediate most neuronal events, and many neurotransmitters are dietary amino acids or their products. Since neuronal function must be carefully controlled, it is imperative that the brain be sealed off from systemically circulating transmitters (eg, glutamic and aspartic acid, norepinephrine, dopamine, and serotonin) and be able to produce its own supply of these transmitters. The brain is sealed off by decreasing the permeability of capillaries throughout the brain and spinal cord so that only ions, water, and necessary small molecules can reach the brain by passive diffusion. Therefore, the blood-brain barrier can be regarded as the tight junctions between specialized endothelial cells of the brain capillaries that prevent the filtration of many small and large charged molecules. It has been suggested that astrocytic processes in contact with capillaries also act as part of the barrier between blood and brain, but their role is still unclear.

The brain capillaries use a number of the uptake mechanisms that have been discussed earlier, such as facilitated diffusion. Since the blood-brain barrier is intended to isolate the neuronal environment from the "contaminated" periphery, the brain circumvents the barrier only to permit entry of the required charged substances that it cannot make itself. For example, there is a competitive and saturable uptake mechanism to permit entry of neutral amino acids (eg, leucine, isoleucine, phenylalanine, and tryptophan). Injection of one inhibits the rate of entry of the others. Most lipid-soluble drugs gain easy access to the brain by simple diffusion, aided by a high rate of blood flow to the brain. The blood-brain barrier blocks the access of many ionized drugs to the brain, however.

The ability of a drug to cross the blood-brain barrier is an important consideration in drug therapy. For example, penicillin does not normally cross the blood-brain barrier. This is fortunate, since penicillin, generally one of the most innocuous drugs when given systemically, is a potent convulsant if it gains access to the brain. Therefore, in meningitis or any condition in which the blood-brain barrier may be damaged, seizures can be expected to result from peripheral penicillin administration. Heroin is more popular than morphine among drug abusers because acetylation of morphine to form heroin increases its lipid solubility and, thus, its rate of passage across the blood-brain barrier into the brain (where it is deacetylated back to morphine), providing a higher concentration of morphine to the regions of the brain that enjoy it. Clinically useful drugs are developed with the blood-brain barrier in mind to either include or eliminate the distribution of the drug to the CNS.

Maternal-Fetal Distribution and Placental Transfer

Like other tissues of the body, the placenta is beautifully suited to its purpose. It is not simply a passive membrane, but a living tissue that synthesizes numerous peptides, enzymes, and hormones; actively transports molecules needed by the fetus; removes catabolites from the fetal circulation; and provides a usually effective immunologic barrier between mother and fetus. It might be presumed that the placenta functions to protect the fetus from many of the solutes in maternal blood much as the blood-brain barrier functions to protect the brain, but this is not the case. Whereas the blood-brain barrier excludes small charged molecules, the placenta allows the bidirectional transfer of most molecules of 600 or less in molecular weight. Since the molecules of the vast majority of drugs are smaller than this limiting size, the optimistic view that the placenta is a barrier to drugs is incorrect. The factors that regulate the entry of molecules into the fetal circulation are the same as those that regulate the passage of molecules across membranes in general. Lipid-soluble drugs diffuse across the placenta passively, and small molecules cross the placental membranes at rates dependent on their molecular weight, charge characteristics, and concentration in the maternal blood.

Research has shown that the placenta contains most of the drug-metabolizing enzymes present in the liver, which suggests that the placenta may be capable of protecting the fetus from some maternal drugs. The placenta cannot demethylate meperidine, however. Although in vitro studies show that the placenta contains enzymes capable of metabolizing drugs, few in vivo data exist to show that the placenta acts as a drug-metabolizing barrier to any significant extent. Little definitive information on the ability of the human fetus to metabolize drugs independently is available, but some basic concepts seem likely. First, the ability of the fetus to metabolize drugs independently is believed to be minimal. Therefore, the elimination of a drug from the fetus is dependent on the maternal plasma drug concentration. As the maternal concentration falls, the drug diffuses from the fetus into the maternal circulation. Second, acutely administered drugs take variable periods of time to reach the fetus in biologically effective concentrations. Thiopental, the highly lipid-soluble barbiturate anesthetic, and alcohol equilibrate within a few minutes of maternal injection, whereas dexamethasone takes hours to equilibrate between maternal and fetal circulations. Therefore, a single dose of a drug may have a profound or minimal effect on the fetus, depending on the drug's absorption, distribution and excretion rates, and the length of time before delivery that the drug is administered. For example, if a patient is given a barbiturate shortly before delivery, the drug may not have enough time to reach a plasma concentration in the fetus high enough to cause drowsiness or respiratory depression after birth. If an anesthetic is given hours before delivery, the fetus may get sufficient drug to cause an undesirable pharmacologic effect. In this case, because the neonate is isolated from the maternal system that removed and metabolized fetal drugs prenatally and because the metabolic capacity of the neonate is minimal, drug action and respiratory depression after delivery might be prolonged. Given the available information, the following conclusions seem warranted:

1. Most, if not all, drugs enter the fetus.
2. The physician cannot determine which fetal drug concentration of which drugs will have an undesirable effect on the fetus.
3. The fetus is a developing organism, and drugs may have effects on the fetus unrelated to their intended clinical purpose; eg, thalidomide is an effective sedative, but is highly teratogenic.
4. The fetus may be able to metabolize certain drugs prenatally, but this cannot be evaluated in vivo by the physician.
5. Caution, when in a state of ignorance, is the approach least likely to produce disastrous consequences.

BIOTRANSFORMATION

As soon as a drug is administered, the body begins to act on it chemically. The chemical reactions that cause biotransformation of drug molecules are mediated by enzymes that originated to transform endogenous substances and environmental compounds to which animals were chronically exposed during their evolutionary development. For example, many biologically active amines in food are normally destroyed by intestinal monoamine oxidase. When monoamine oxidase is inhibited pharmacologically, the tyramine in cheese, wine, and fermented products is not destroyed and can increase blood pressure to a dangerous level by an indirect sympathomimetic effect. The two separate classes of drug-metabolizing enzymes are the microsomal and the nonmicrosomal enzymes.

First-Pass Effect

An interesting feature of GI function is the first-pass effect. The blood supply to most of the intestine goes to the liver via the portal circulation before entering the systemic venous circulation. This gives the liver an opportunity to destroy harmful exogenous substances before they reach the general circulation. Nitroglycerin, for example, is generally not given orally, since a large proportion of the administered dose is metabolized in one pass through the liver. This first-pass effect plays an important role in the use of many orally administered drugs. As mentioned previously, however, the blood flow to the oral mucosa and the rectum avoids the portal circulation; therefore, drugs given by the sublingual and rectal routes are not subjected to a first-pass effect.

Microsomal and Nonmicrosomal Drug Metabolism

The term *microsomal* does not refer to a particular cellular organelle. The microsomes are a centrifugation fraction prepared from liver or other tissues that contains the smooth endoplasmic reticulum and the enzymes associated with the reticular membranes. These enzymes are normally involved in the biotransformation of steroid hormones, fatty acids, and bilirubin, as well as in the metabolism of natural environmental and dietary contaminants. In addition, the microsomal enzymes catalyze glucuronide conjugations, most of the oxidation reactions involving drugs, and some reductions and hydrolyses.

Two unique properties distinguish microsomal from nonmicrosomal enzymes. First, microsomal enzymes accept primarily lipid-soluble substrates. This is probably because these enzymes are membrane-associated and the ability of a substrate to interact with the lipid membrane is a required condition for reaction. Second, and more importantly, the activity of the microsomal enzymes can be greatly affected by prior or concomitant treatment with drugs.

Nonmicrosomal enzymes, which are present in plasma, intestine, liver, and other tissues, catalyze all conjugation reactions except glucuronide conjugations. Hydrolyses and some oxidation and reduction reactions are also catalyzed by nonmicrosomal enzymes. These enzymes catalyze reactions involving substrates from two basic sources: 1) parent drugs (eg, aspirin or sulfonamides), which are metabolized directly to more water-soluble conjugates, and 2) the products of microsomal drug metabolism. Unlike the substrates of the microsomal enzymes, the substrates of nonmicrosomal enzymes are not necessarily lipid-soluble. Furthermore, prior exposure to drugs does not affect the activity of nonmicrosomal enzymes as it affects the activity of the microsomal enzymes. Both microsomal and nonmicrosomal enzymes can vary in activity between individuals, however, and these differences can greatly affect the rate at which an individual metabolizes a particular drug.

Types of Reactions

SYNTHETIC REACTIONS

The synthetic reactions of the body that alter a drug structurally involve the joining of the drug molecule with a chemical supplied by the body. For such a reaction, a drug must have a chemical group capable of forming a conjugate. These groups include the hydroxyl (-OH), amino ($-NH_2$), carboxyl (-COOH), and sulfhydryl (-SH) groups. All conjugation reactions, except glucuronidation, are catalyzed by nonmicrosomal enzymes.

Acylation. In acylation, the conjugation of an amino acid (eg, glycine or glutamine) with the carboxyl group of a drug molecule forms a generally more water-soluble conjugate that is more readily excreted in the urine. For example,

$$\overset{\displaystyle O}{\underset{\displaystyle \|}{}}\qquad\qquad\qquad\overset{\displaystyle O}{\underset{\displaystyle \|}{}}$$
$$RCOOH - RC\text{-}S\text{-}CoA + NH_2CH_2COOH \rightarrow RCNHCH_2COOH + CoA\text{-}SH$$

Acetylation. The conjugation of an acid supplied by the body (eg, acetic acid) with the amino (-NH$_2$) group of the drug to form an acetylated derivative (-NH-CO-CH$_3$) is acetylation.

$$\overset{\displaystyle O}{\underset{\displaystyle \|}{}}\qquad\qquad\overset{\displaystyle O}{\underset{\displaystyle \|}{}}$$
$$RNH_2 + CH_3C\text{-}S\text{-}CoA \rightarrow RNHCCH_3 + CoA\text{-}SH$$

Methylation. The process by which a methyl group (-CH$_3$), usually derived from the amino acid methionine, is transferred to a ring-associated hydroxyl group, to amino groups (-NH$_2$), or to a nitrogen molecule within a ring is methylation. These methylation reactions are commonly used by the body to synthesize and catabolize many endogenous substances, as well as drugs. Examples include the catabolism of catecholamine transmitters, ie, norepinephrine, epinephrine, and dopamine, as well as the methylation of nicotinamide to *N*-methyl-nicotinamide. Methylation frequently increases the lipid solubility of a compound, but it can also result in a charged nitrogen molecule that is more water-soluble and, therefore, more likely to be excreted by the kidney, eg, the aforementioned nicotinamide conversion to the quaternary ammonium compound *N*-methyl-nicotinamide.

$$R\text{-}XH + S\text{-adenosylmethionine} \rightarrow R\text{-}X\text{-}CH_3$$
$$+ \; S\text{-adenosylhomocysteine} \; (X = O, S, \text{or } N)$$

Sulfate Conjugation. Ethereal sulfate formation involves the transfer of a sulfate group derived from cystine, for example, to the hydroxyl group of a drug.

$$ROH + 3'\text{-phosphoadenosine} - 5'\text{-phosphosulfate} \rightarrow$$
$$\overset{\displaystyle O}{\underset{\displaystyle \|}{}}$$
$$RO\text{-}S\text{-}OH + 3'\text{-phosphoadenosine} - 5'\text{-phosphate}$$
$$\underset{\displaystyle O}{\overset{\displaystyle \|}{}}$$

Glucuronide Formation. Glucuronidation is a common reaction in drug metabolism and involves the conjugation of a molecule of glucuronic acid ($C_6H_9O_6$), derived from glucose, with the appropriate functional group of the drug. The functional groups available for glucuronidation include amino (-NH$_2$), carboxyl (-COOH), hydroxyl (-OH), and sulfhydryl (-SH) groups. Because glucuronides are highly charged compounds, they are excreted in the urine. Glucuronides are also excreted in the bile. Bacterial enzymes in the intestine often cleave the glucuronide linkage, however, so that the parent drug can be released. If the liberated drug can be absorbed, this process of absorption, elimination, cleavage, and reabsorption is termed *enterohepatic circulation.* This can prevent the excretion of the drug and prolong its action in the body.

$$C_6H_9O_6 - UDP + R\text{-}OH \rightarrow C_6H_9O_6\text{-}O\text{-}R + UDP$$

UDP-glucuronic acid

NONSYNTHETIC REACTIONS

In nonsynthetic reactions, the parent drug is transformed by hydrolysis, oxidation, or reduction. This generally yields a less lipid-soluble molecule that is then often conjugated by one of the synthetic reactions already discussed. These first-stage biotransformations can be catalyzed by either nonmicrosomal or microsomal enzymes.

Hydrolysis. A hydrolytic reaction involves the cleavage of an ester or amide linkage by an esterase or an amidase, respectively. Therefore, the products of an esterase-mediated reaction are an alcohol and an acid; the products of an amidase reaction, an amine and an acid. Drugs such as procaine, aspirin, cocaine, meperidine, and atropine are hydrolyzed. Esterases, found in plasma, liver, and many other tissues, are nonmicrosomal (not in the microsomal centrifugation fraction). Amidases are primarily of hepatic origin.

$$\begin{array}{ccc} O & & O \\ \| & & \| \\ R\text{-}C\text{-}OR' + H_2O & \rightarrow & R\text{-}C\text{-}OH + R'\text{-}OH \end{array}$$

esterase

$$\begin{array}{ccc} O & & O \\ \| & & \| \\ R\text{-}C\text{-}N\text{-}R' + H_2O & \rightarrow & R\text{-}C\text{-}OH + R'NH_2 \end{array}$$

amidase

Oxidation. A large proportion of drug biotransformations are accomplished by oxidation. Such reactions can be catalyzed by microsomal and nonmicrosomal enzymes. These reactions include

1. Oxidation of aromatic rings by addition of a hydroxyl group

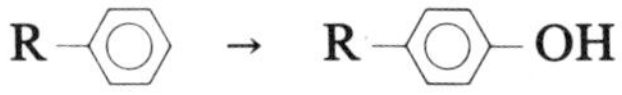

$$R-\bigcirc \rightarrow R-\bigcirc-OH$$

2. Oxidation of alkyl chains

$$R\text{-}CH_2OH \rightarrow R\overset{O}{\underset{\|}{C}}\text{-}H \rightarrow R\overset{O}{\underset{\|}{C}}\text{-}OH$$

3. Oxidative dealkylation

$R\text{-}OCH_3 \rightarrow R\text{-}OH + CH_2O$
O-dealkylation, or
$R\text{-}NHCH_3 \rightarrow RNH_2 + CH_2O$
N-dealkylation

4. *N*-oxidation

$$RNH_2 \rightarrow RNO_2$$

5. Sulfoxidation

$$R\text{-}S\text{-}R' \rightarrow R\overset{O}{\underset{\|}{S}}\text{-}R'$$

6. Desulfuration

$$R\text{-}SH \rightarrow R\text{-}OH$$

7. Deamination

$$R\text{-}NH_2 \rightarrow R\overset{O}{\underset{\|}{C}}\text{-}H$$

Alterations in the Rate of Drug Metabolism

INHIBITION OF DRUG METABOLISM

The rate at which a drug is metabolized often determines its concentration at the receptor site and the duration of its action. Factors that decrease the rate of drug metabolism are clinically relevant, since a diminished drug-metabolizing capacity makes it necessary for the clinician to adjust the dosage. This is particularly important for drugs that have a low therapeutic index, ie, the toxic dose is close to the effective dose. The three main factors that inhibit the rate of drug metabolism are genetic influences, disease processes, and drug interactions.

Genetic Influences. Since the synthesis of the enzymes that metabolize drugs involves gene transcription and translation, genetically different individuals exhibit differences in their rate of drug metabolism. The genetic component has been demonstrated in studies of twins; monozygotic twins exhibit very similar drug-metabolizing capacities, while dizygotic twins differ in their drug-metabolizing capacity to a greater extent.

Genetically determined differences in drug metabolic rates are responsible for some of the clinically observed differences in patient response to a given drug. For example, the depolarizing neuromuscular junction blocker succinylcholine is used as a muscle relaxant during surgery. Most individuals possess a plasma cholinesterase that rapidly metabolizes succinylcholine, but some patients have an atypical, abnormal enzyme that does not metabolize succinylcholine at a normal rate. These patients can exhibit prolonged apnea due to respiratory paralysis when given succinylcholine. Genetic factors may also result in the slow acetylation of hydralazine, isoniazid, and procainamide (which can lead to a lupuslike syndrome) and sensitivity to phenytoin and bishydroxycoumarin due to slow hepatic metabolism. These genetic influences are particularly important when the drug has a low therapeutic index.

Disease Processes. The rate of drug metabolism will obviously be decreased when the drug-metabolizing cells of the liver or other tissues have been destroyed. Hepatic necrosis, which occurs in many diseases, requires a reduction in dosage of many drugs normally metabolized by the liver.

Drug Interactions. Because the microsomal enzymes are not usually saturated with substrate, most reactions are first-order (reaction rates dependent on substrate concentration). In this situation, two substrates for the same enzyme do not have significant competitive inhibitory effects, since the enzyme capacity is sufficient for both drugs to be metabolized simultaneously. Some drugs are metabolized by zero-order reactions, however, in which the reaction rate is independent of substrate concentration. The anticonvulsant phenytoin and the anticoagulant bishydroxy-coumarin, for example, inhibit each other's metabolism, since enzyme capacity is not sufficient to metabolize both simultaneously. In addition, the rate of metabolism of some drugs, eg, lidocaine, is dependent on the rate at which they are delivered to the metabolic enzymes by blood flow. Therefore, any treatment or disease process that interferes with hepatic blood flow could inhibit the rate of metabolism of one of these drugs. This is not a common problem, however, and the rate of metabolism of most drugs does not depend on hepatic blood flow.

INDUCTION OF MICROSOMAL DRUG METABOLISM

The fact that some drugs greatly increase the activity and amount of drug-metabolizing enzymes is of considerable clinical importance. Two main types of compounds induce microsomal enzymes. Phenobarbital and some drugs that resemble phenobarbital structurally increase the synthesis of one set of drug-metabolizing microsomal enzymes; the polycyclic hydrocarbons increase the synthesis of another set. The available evidence indicates that the increase in enzymatic activity is due to a stimulation of protein synthesis associated with increases in the amount of smooth endoplasmic reticulum and in liver weight.

The induction of microsomal enzyme activity can produce important clinical effects. Phenobarbital, for example, can increase the rate of drug metabolism not only of phenobarbital itself, but also of many other drugs. One well-known example is the combination of phenobarbital, used chronically as an antiepileptic, and bishydroxycoumarin, an anticoagulant. When bishydroxycoumarin is given alone, a particular dose increases the prothrombin time (an index of coagulation) to the desired extent. If phenobarbital is given concurrently, the rate of metabolism of the anticoagulant increases, resulting in a decrease in the anticoagulant concentration after a given dose. Therefore, the dose of bishydroxycoumarin must be increased in order to produce the desired anticoagulant effect. Once a maintenance dose of bishydroxycoumarin has been established, cessation of phenobarbital treatment decreases the rate of microsomal metabolism toward the normal range, resulting in a bishydroxycoumarin concentration that could produce hemorrhage.

Drug Metabolism and Drug Toxicity

Microsomal drug metabolism can result in the formation of both toxic and nontoxic metabolites. Acetaminophen, for example, is normally metabolized in a two-step reaction. In the first step, a highly reactive intermediate is formed; in the second step, this intermediate is normally combined with glutathione to form a harmless product. When 6 g or more of acetaminophen is ingested, the reactive intermediate is formed and reacted with glutathione at a rate that exceeds the liver's ability to make glutathione. In this case, the reactive intermediate N-acetyl-p-benzoquinone accumulates, binds to liver cells, and causes liver necrosis, coma, and death.

It has also been suggested that induction of microsomal drug metabolism by polycyclic hydrocarbons results in the accumulation of highly reactive intermediates of drugs and environmental chemicals that bind to DNA and may be carcinogenic.

EXCRETION

There are a limited number of routes out of the body. The routes of perspiration, lacrimation, salivation, and ejaculation are quantitatively unimportant for drugs. The respiratory route is a significant excretion route for volatile anesthetics, but the main routes of excretion for drugs are the feces and urine.

The feces contain unabsorbed drug, drug that has been secreted into the saliva and then swallowed, drug metabolites formed as a result of bacterial biotransformation within the gut, and drug metabolites formed as a result of hepatic drug metabolism and secretion into the bile. Through the enterohepatic circulation, many compounds secreted into the bile are reabsorbed into the blood and excreted via the single most important route for drug elimination—the kidney.

A drug or drug metabolite can pass from blood to urine by glomerular filtration or tubular secretion; furthermore, it can pass from urine back to blood by active or passive tubular reabsorption. The mechanism for active transport in the proximal tubule normally transports uric acid and other endogenous products. Exogenous acids, such as penicillin, can be transported into the urine by the same carrier mechanism. Since the tubular secretion of penicillin terminates its action, the acid transport inhibitor probenecid can be used to prolong therapeutic plasma concentrations of penicillin by inhibiting competitively its secretion into the urine. Similarly, the active reabsorption of uric acid can be blocked by probenecid when it is desirable to increase the rate of uric acid excretion (as in gout).

Passive reabsorption of molecules from urine to blood is determined by the relative lipid/water solubility of the drug. Although filtered into the urine, highly lipid-soluble drugs are reabsorbed. The properties of absorption described previously apply to renal reabsorption of weak acids and bases. For example, since only the uncharged molecules of the weak base amphetamine are passively reabsorbed, the rate of amphetamine excretion in the urine can be increased by acidifying the urine to shift the chemical equilibrium in the direction of the charged form of amphetamine. The amphetamine filtered into the urine is then predominantly charged and, therefore, trapped and excreted in the urine. Similarly, the urinary excretion rate of the weak acid salicylate can be greatly increased by alkalinizing the urine.

DRUG-RECEPTOR INTERACTIONS

One of the most basic concepts in pharmacology is that a physiologic process can be altered by the influence of a chemical on a cellular constituent (receptor) that is in some way related to the physiological process. Therefore, a drug cannot impart entirely new functions to a cell, but can act only to modulate cell function and activity.

Defined in its broadest sense, a receptor is simply the physical entity with which a drug molecule interacts to produce a pharmacologic effect. Therefore, a heavy metal ion could be regarded as a receptor for the chelator used to treat toxic reactions to a heavy metal. For the vast majority of drugs, however, the receptor is considered a normal cellular constituent that is in some way directly related to a physiological process. The major category of receptors and the best examples to use to illustrate the drug-receptor interaction are proteins that mediate normal biologic responses. These proteins exhibit a three-dimensional shape in space and a unique set of charge characteristics, both of which can change after they bind a molecule for which they have chemical affinity. The change in receptor configuration can alter membrane permeability to ions if the receptor is linked to an ion channel, or it can result in translocation of the receptor from one part of the cell to another, where it produces a biologic effect (as in the case of a cytoplasmic steroid receptor).

A drug is called an *agonist* if its action on the receptor is similar to the action of an endogenous ligand that evokes a biologic response. A drug is termed an *antagonist* if it prevents the receptor from mediating a biologic response. An antagonist can act competitively by binding to the active site in such a manner that the access of an agonist to the active site is blocked, or it can act noncompetitively to block the biologic response. If the receptor is an enzyme and the biologic response is the formation of product, a noncompetitive antagonist could 1) bind to the active site irreversibly, thus preventing any agonist-receptor interaction; 2) bind to an area other than the active site, thus changing the three-dimensional configuration of the receptor and rendering the enzyme inactive; 3) chelate a needed cofactor without ever coming in contact with the enzyme; or 4) bind chemically to anything that, in any way, protects the substrate from enzymatic attack.

In the most restricted sense, the term *receptor* is not used to describe an enzyme, but to describe an entity that binds a ligand, undergoes a conformational change, and then causes a change in the adjacent membrane. In this narrow definition of the word *receptor*, the receptor is a protein consisting of amino acids with different charge and steric characteristics. When the protein assumes its "resting" three-dimensional configuration, a particular combination of amino acid groups determines the chemical qualities of the "active" or binding site of the molecule. The charge and physical shape of the active site presumably bind the endogenous ligand optimally (from a biologic, not chemical view) and bind exogenous compounds with greater or lesser avidity.

The exact way in which a ligand and a receptor interact to combine and then produce a biologic response remains a subject of conjecture. The general view is that the ligand binds to the receptor by a combination of ionic, hydrogen, and Van der Waals bonds and, in some cases (eg, phenoxybenzamine), covalent bonds. The ligand binding is believed to change the charge characteristics of the receptor in such a way that its three-dimensional configuration changes. This configurational alteration initiates changes in characteristics, such as membrane permeability and fluidity, that cause a subsequent change in cellular function. Standard pharmacology texts should be consulted for detailed discussions of the subject.

Dose-Response Relationship

A basic tenet of pharmacology is that, within some range of drug concentrations, the evoked biologic reponse is proportional to the concentration of drug at its receptor site and the number of receptor sites available to bind drug. At any drug concentration below that necessary to produce an effect, a small increase in drug concentration has little effect. As the concentration approaches the effective range, an increase in the dose increases the magnitude of the response. As the available receptor sites become occupied or the maximal activity of the process is reached, a further increase in drug concentration has little effect on the response. When plotted on a graph, a dose *v* response curve takes an S shape (Fig 1–1). This type of curve is useful to illustrate the concepts of potency *v* efficacy and agonism *v* antagonism.

Different drugs that are able to induce the same effect are said to have equal efficacy. The drugs may vary in potency, however, which means that it takes less of one drug to produce the same effect (Fig 1–2). Differences in potency most likely reflect differences in the way the drugs are absorbed, distributed, metabolized, and excreted, rather than differences in their mechanisms of action. Differences in potency would be important if the drugs varied greatly in price, but efficacy, not the amount of chemical needed, is important in therapy.

Figure 1–3 shows differences in both efficacy and potency. It may also be helpful to consider a real example. The hallucinogen lysergic acid diethylamide (LSD) is extremely potent; only a very small amount (< 100 μg) is needed to produce an hallucinogenic state. Mescaline produces a nearly identical hallucinogenic state, but 4,000 times more mescaline is required to do so (approximately 350 mg). Therefore, mescaline is said to be as efficacious as LSD, but much less potent. This difference in potency is relatively unimportant, because the two drugs

Fig 1–1. *Typical dose-response curve. At a dose so low that the drug concentration at the receptor site does not produce a biologic response, increasing the dose slightly has negligible effects (A). As the dose is increased further, the slope of curve (B) indicates the affinity with which the receptor interacts with the drug. If affinity is high, the slope is likely to be steep; a small increase in drug concentration produces a marked increase in the rate of drug-receptor interactions. Once a maximal response is produced, a further increase in dose produces no greater response (C).*

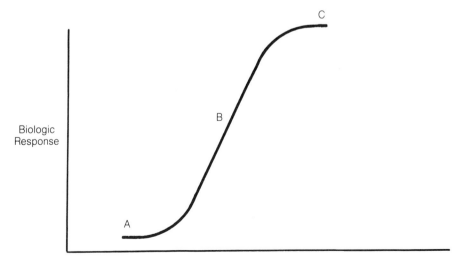

Biologic Response

Log Dose

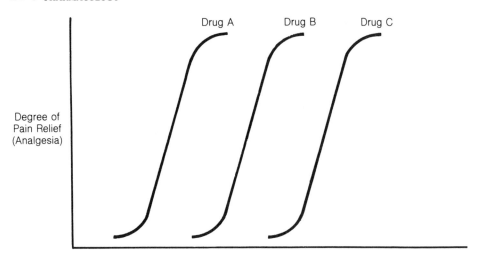

Fig 1–2. *Differences in drug potency of three analgesics. Since drugs A, B, and C produce similar responses (similar slopes and maximal responses), they probably produce their effects by interaction at the same receptor. They differ only in terms of potency.*

Fig 1–3. *Differences in efficacy and potency of three drugs. Similar responses of drugs Y and Z suggest that they act by the same mechanism, but they differ in potency. Because drug X produces a greater maximal response, it is said to be more efficacious.*

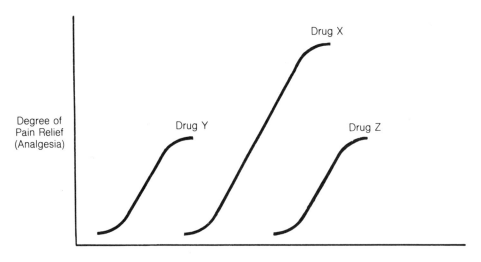

produce the same result (hallucinations). Efficacy is primarily a reflection of the relationship between a drug and its receptor. Differences in efficacy suggest differences in the mechanisms by which drugs evoke biologic responses.

Dose-response curves can also be used to illustrate competitive and noncompetitive antagonism. In competitive antagonism, an antagonist competes for the same active site on the receptor as does an agonist. An antagonist shifts the dose-response curve for the agonist to the right and a higher dose of antagonist shifts the curve further to the right (Fig 1–4). The way in which the antagonist shifts the curve provides information on how the two drugs interact. In competitive antagonism, the curves are parallel and of similar shape, ie, the antagonist does not prevent the maximal effect of the agonist; however, more agonist must be used to produce the maximal effect. In noncompetitive antagonism, the antagonist prevents the maximal effect of the agonist, regardless of how much agonist is present (Fig 1–5). If both drugs interacted with the same receptor in a similar manner, the agonist would still be able to produce the same maximal response at higher doses. Curves showing noncompetitive antagonism do not provide information about how the antagonism is produced or suggest actions at different receptors. Indeed, two drugs could interact with the same receptor; one could bind to the receptor, thus preventing the other drug from interacting with it.

Fig 1–4. *Competitive antagonism. Biologic responses evoked by drug X vary according to dose of drug Y. Since more of drug X is needed to produce a similar response when drug Y is present, drug Y is an antagonist of drug X. Drug X produces the same maximal response, only at a higher dose, and the curves are parallel; therefore, drug Y is said to be a competitive antagonist, probably competing with drug X for the same receptors.*

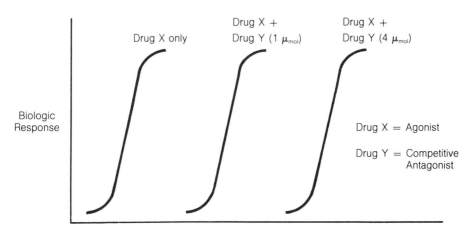

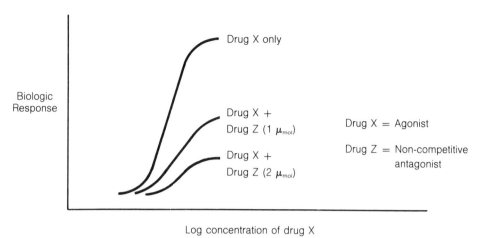

Fig 1–5. *Noncompetitive antagonism. Drug Z changes the maximal response that drug X can evoke, regardless of the dose of drug X, as well as the slopes of the curves.*

Selectivity *v* Specificity

The terms *selectivity* and *specificity* are often misused. A drug has specificity if all its pharmacologic effects result from a single type of drug-receptor interaction, regardless of how many effects it produces. For example, isoproterenol interacts with β-adrenergic receptors, but has little affinity for α-adrenergic receptors. Epinephrine has an affinity for both receptors. Therefore, isoproterenol is more specific than epinephrine in relation to adrenergic receptors. A drug is said to be selective if it produces only the biologic response intended. For example, the cholinergic agonist methacholine produces many effects after injection (eg, salivation, lacrimation, urination, and diarrhea), but all are caused by an interaction with similar muscarinic cholinergic receptors. Therefore, methacholine is said to be relatively specific (it acts primarily on one type of receptor), but not selective (it produces many effects). Penicillin is a relatively specific drug (it acts primarily on bacterial cell wall synthesis) that is also selective (it produces few effects other than its antibacterial action). Clearly, selectivity and specificity are important considerations in pharmacologic therapy in order to decrease the occurrence of unwanted side-effects.

Therapeutic Index

Each drug produces a therapeutic effect and, usually at higher doses, a toxic effect. By comparing the lethal dose in 50% of an animal population receiving the drug (LD_{50}) or the toxic dose in 50% of the patient population (TD_{50}) with the effective dose in 50% of the population (ED_{50}), it is possible to arrive at a therapeutic index for each drug $\left(\dfrac{LD_{50}}{ED_{50}} \text{ or } \dfrac{TD_{50}}{ED_{50}}\right)$. This ratio indicates the margin between the therapeutic dose and the toxic dose. For a drug with a very large therapeutic index, such as penicillin, there is little risk of toxic effects at therapeutic doses. For a drug with a low therapeutic index, such as digitalis, the clinician must carefully monitor drug dosage, plasma concentration, and therapeutic effect because the toxic dose is very close to the therapeutic dose.

PHARMACOKINETICS

Historically, it has been necessary for the clinician to rely solely on observation of the patient to determine the therapeutic efficacy of a particular drug treatment. Now, however, analytical methods are available that enable the clinician to correlate the presence of drug in the body fluids or compartments with the observed biologic effects of the drug. Although the effects of some drugs long outlast their presence in the body, most drugs cease to produce effects after they have been eliminated from the body. For these drugs, measurement of plasma drug concentration at intervals after injection can provide information about how the body handles a drug. The relatively recent development of the field of pharmacokinetics should be viewed as an adjunctive means of evaluation, not as a replacement for clinical observation.

Plasma Decay Curve

If the plasma concentration of a drug is measured every minute, from immediately after injection to days after injection, and the values are plotted on a logarithmic graph *v* time, a typical two-phase plasma decay curve is obtained (Fig 1–6). As the drug distributes throughout the blood and into rapidly perfused tissues of the body, the plasma drug concentration falls rapidly until a particular concentration is reached. This initial process is called the distribution phase or α-phase. The plasma concentration of the drug then begins to fall at a slower rate, usually reflecting the rate at which the drug is eliminated from the body. This latter phase is called the elimination phase or β-phase. If a drug's plasma concentration reflects its concentration at the site of action, a plasma decay curve can provide information about the effectiveness of the treatment and the rate at which the drug must be given to maintain a therapeutic concentration.

Pharmacokinetic principles require that the body be conceptualized in terms of compartments. The blood is referred to as the central compartment. When equilibrium is reached between the drug in the blood and the drug in the tissues, the main process acting to decrease plasma concentration further, albeit at a slower

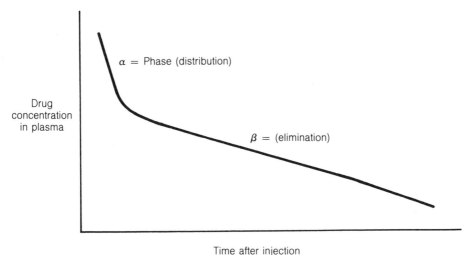

Fig 1–6. *Typical two-phase plasma decay curve.*

rate, is elimination of the drug. The curve plotted as a result of distribution and elimination is said to fit a two-compartment model. If blood samples are not taken until after the brief tissue distribution phase is complete, the plasma decay curve is usually a straight line, reflecting the rate at which the drug is eliminated from the body. In this case, the data are said to fit a one-compartment model; ie, the drug in plasma is already in equilibrium with the drug in tissues by the time blood samples are first taken, and the entire body acts as a single compartment from which the drug is removed.

The plasma kinetics of most drugs fit a two-compartment model, but several drugs exhibit three distinct phases on a plasma decay curve (Fig 1–7) and more could no doubt be demonstrated if an infinite number of blood samples were taken before, during, and after injection. Strong binding of drug to a "deep" compartment, eg, bone or fat, results in a third or γ-phase. In this case, there is little net efflux of drug from the deep compartment until the plasma drug concentration falls to a certain point. Then, return of drug from the deep compartment into the blood constitutes the third phase.

It is important to note that any plasma decay curve is simply a graphic plot of numbers obtained from analyses of fluid samples. The appearance of a third or γ-phase does not automatically indicate the return of a drug from the deep compartment. The anticoagulant bishydroxycoumarin, for example, exhibits three plasma phases that have been interpreted as 1) a blood distribution phase, 2) a separate tissue distribution phase, and 3) an elimination phase. The appearance of three phases indicates only that three separate kinetic phases exist. What a particular phase represents in meaningful biologic terms is an inference drawn by the investigator.

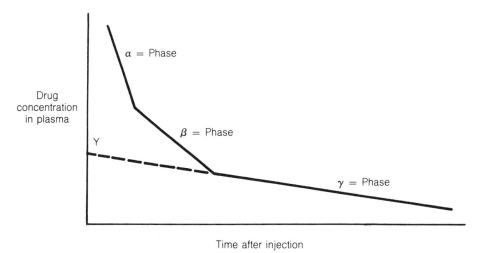

Fig 1–7. *Plasma decay curve described by three-compartment model. Drug concentration at zero time is indicated by Y.*

Half-Life

The plasma half-life of a drug is the period of time required for the plasma drug concentration to be halved. Because the plasma drug concentration does not parallel the drug concentration at its receptor site in all cases, it cannot automatically be assumed that plasma drug data provide information about the desired biologic effect of a drug. For a large number of drugs, however, plasma decay curves do reflect the biologic response, and plasma half-life data yield useful information about drug action. Half-life can be calculated from the terminal portion of a plasma decay curve according to the following formula:

$$t_{\frac{1}{2}} = \frac{0.693}{\beta}$$

where $t_{\frac{1}{2}}$ is the half-life and β is the slope of the elimination phase.

Three points about half-lives merit emphasis. First, the overall rate of elimination of a drug from the body is independent of the dose administered, since, in the vast majority of cases, drug elimination is a first-order process. Second, the terminal portion of the plasma decay curve used to calculate the elimination rate constant has the same slope, regardless of the route of administration, as long as absorption and distribution are complete. Third, the half-life of a drug may be affected by any factor that affects the rates of metabolism or excretion. Differences in drug metabolism usually underlie the differences in drug half-lives among individuals. Similarly, disease processes, particularly those affecting hepatic or renal function, greatly affect the half-life of a drug that is metabolized and excreted by these routes. Altered rates of elimination are of paramount interest clinically in determining the correct dose when a therapeutic concentration of a drug must be maintained over time.

Calculation of the Volume of Distribution

The apparent volume of distribution (Vd_a) can be calculated from the plasma decay curve. Extension of the elimination phase of the curve back to the origin on the Y axis yields a point (Fig 1–7) that represents the theoretical plasma concentration obtained immediately after the total dose was administered before any excretion occurred, assuming that distribution occurred instantaneously. Dividing the total dose administered by the plasma concentration at zero time yields the apparent volume of distribution.

Clearance

The rate of elimination of a drug from the body can be expressed as clearance (C):

$$C = \beta Vd_a = \frac{Vd_a \times 0.693}{t_{1/2}}$$

or

$$t_{1/2} = \frac{0.693}{C} \times Vd_a$$

The clearance value is expressed in units of volume/time. For a drug that is excreted primarily by the kidney, for example, the renal clearance value (in ml/min) refers simply to the volume of blood that is cleared of a drug by the kidney in 1 minute. An individual with normal renal function filters approximately 120 ml blood every minute. Some compounds (eg, creatinine, inulin, and mannitol) are excreted into the urine solely by glomerular filtration and are not reabsorbed. Since 120 ml blood are filtered every minute, a normal subject has 120 ml blood cleared of creatinine every minute. The renal clearance value is often used to tailor an individual dosage schedule for a patient with renal impairment.

Different solutes have different clearance values. A clearance value of 600 ml/min, does not mean that 600 ml blood are filtered every minute, but that 600 ml blood are cleared of drug every minute. This reflects the glomerular filtration plus active secretion of drug into the urine. A compound that is reabsorbed after filtration, eg, glucose, has a zero clearance value, since it is not excreted and, therefore, no blood has been cleared of glucose.

Clearance studies with compounds known to be handled in a certain way by the body can be used to test kidney function and to provide information about the body's handling of a drug. Generally speaking, a renal clearance value of approximately 120 ml/min reflects glomerular filtration. A higher value reflects both filtration and secretion; a lower value, filtration and reabsorption. The renal clearance (C_R) can be calculated from urinary solute measurement according to the formula:

$$C_R = \frac{UV}{P}$$

where U is the urinary concentration of drug or other solute in mg/ml, V is the number of milliliters of urine excreted per minute, and P is the concentration of drug or solute in plasma (in mg/ml).

DRUG INTERACTIONS

Drugs are often given in combination. Since many different processes govern the way in which a particular drug is handled by the body, any drug or disease that alters one or more of these processes can affect the pharmacologic disposition of that drug. Liver disease greatly affects the plasma concentration of a hepatically metabolized drug, and renal failure does the same for renally excreted drugs, necessitating a reduction of drug dosage. Unfortunately, drug interactions are often unexpected and difficult to evaluate; furthermore, the mechanism of the interaction may be unknown.

Interactions at the Absorption Site

Since the absorption of a drug is dependent on its solubility, its charged/uncharged nature, and the length of time it is in the GI tract, any drug that affects these variables can change the rate of another's absorption. For example, orally administered iron combines with tetracyclines to form an insoluble complex. Because a drug must be in solution to be absorbed, neither the tetracycline nor the iron is absorbed if they are administered together. Similarly, cholestyramine resin binds cholesterol to prevent its absorption, but it also binds a variety of other drugs, including warfarin and digoxin. Anticholinergic drugs decrease stomach emptying. Therefore, these compounds decrease the absorption rate of drugs that are absorbed from the small intestine and increase the absorption rate of drugs that are normally poorly absorbed because of rapid transit.

Interactions as a Result of Altered Plasma Protein Binding

There are two main ways in which one drug can change the plasma protein binding of another. One drug can displace another by competition for the binding site. The displacement of warfarin by phenylbutazone, for example, results in possibly hemorrhagic concentrations of free warfarin. A drug can also change the number of binding sites available to another drug. For example, estradiol increases the concentration of plasma proteins that bind glucocorticoids and iodine; therefore, women who take oral contraceptives have high protein-bound iodine levels in the absence of hyperthyroidism.

Interactions at the Site of Drug Action

A drug can compete with another drug at the site of action to potentiate or inhibit the effect of the other drug. For example, tricyclic antidepressants inhibit the neuronal uptake mechanism by which guanethidine enters the nerve terminal. Since guanethidine must enter the sympathetic nerve terminal in order to exert its antihypertensive effects, tricyclics inhibit the antihypertensive activity of guanethidine. A more common type of interaction occurs at the receptor itself between two agonists or between an agonist and an antagonist. For example, methacholine is a muscarinic cholinergic of the urinary bladder in postsurgical atony. The concomitant use of atropine for bronchial congestion would result in competitive inhibition of methacholine's effect since both drugs produce their respective pharmacologic effects by interacting with the same type of receptor.

Interactions at the Site of Metabolism

A commonly encountered form of drug interaction occurs at the site of metabolism. Many drugs are metabolized by the hepatic mixed function oxidase system, and any drug that affects this system produces a marked effect on the plasma concentrations of drugs metabolized by this system. Induction of drug metabolism by barbiturates, rifampin, or phenytoin will decrease the plasma concentrations of many drugs. This increased rate of drug metabolism is a common cause of therapeutic failure with steroids, such as oral contraceptives, since steroids are metabolized by the membrane-bound microsomal enzymes. Increased rates of drug metabolism also decrease the effect of β-blockers, antidepressants, anticoagulants, digitoxin, tetracyclines, phenothiazines, and many other drugs. Conversely, inhibition of microsomal enzymes by cimetidine, disulfiram, chloramphenicol, and metronidazole increases the plasma concentrations of a variety of drugs. Therefore, drug-induced changes in the rates of drug metabolism can make a normally effective treatment an ineffective treatment or even an overdose. This type of drug interaction is actually the basis for the use of disulfiram, which inhibits the metabolism of ethanol to acetate by blocking the degradation of acetaldehyde. Since the accumulation of acetaldehyde is phenomenally unpleasant, alcoholics who take disulfiram risk an expected and miserable drug interaction should they succumb to the temptation. Other drug interactions, such as the decrease in oral contraceptive effect caused by ampicillin or the decrease in gua-nethidine effect caused by oral contraceptives, have been observed, although no rational reason for the clinical observation has been found. The two points to remember are 1) that interactions are common and should be anticipated, and 2) that many interactions can be evaluated by monitoring the plasma concentrations and kinetics of drugs.

Interactions at the Site of Excretion

The primary excretion site for drug interactions is the kidney. Renally excreted drugs enter the urine by glomerular filtration and active tubular secretion. They reenter the blood from the urine by active tubular absorption and by passive diffusion. Therefore, any drug that affects any of these processes alters the rate of excretion of other drugs. Drug interactions can be used to advantage, for example, to increase the rate of excretion of an unwanted drug; after amphetamine or phencyclidine overdose, acidification of the urine with ammonium chloride or ascorbic acid favors the charged form of amphetamine or phencyclidine, thereby decreasing the rate of reabsorption.

2
Sedatives and Hypnotics

Benzodiazepines
  Mechanism of Action
  Pharmacokinetics
  Adverse Effects
Barbiturates
  Mechanism of Action
  Pharmacokinetics
  Adverse Effects

It is necessary to understand how neurons work together to maintain the normal state in order to understand how centrally acting drugs produce their effects. The regulation of neuronal activity within the normal range of brain function can be viewed, in part, as a balance between excitatory and inhibitory events. Virtually all neurons receive a multitude of excitatory and inhibitory inputs and, in turn, form many connections with other neurons. Neurons do not communicate by physical contacts, but by the release of chemical neurotransmitters that change the postsynaptic cell's permeability to certain ions; in this way, "information" is transferred from one cell to the next. The postsynaptic cell usually passes on this information to another cell, but it can also excite or inhibit the first cell by a feedback mechanism.

Whether a cell excites or inhibits another cell depends primarily on whether it releases an intrinsically excitatory or inhibitory neurotransmitter. The most common excitatory neurotransmitters are acetylcholine and the amino acids aspartate and glutamate. The main inhibitory neurotransmitters in the brain and spinal cord are γ-aminobutyric acid (GABA) and the amino acid glycine, respectively.

An explanation of the maintenance of a proper neuronal balance between excitatory and inhibitory mechanisms was developed by Eccles and co-workers in the 1950s. According to their now generally accepted view, excitatory cells activate inhibitory interneurons that feedback-inhibit the excitatory cells. For example, when a stimulus induces a spinal motor neuron to fire, a corresponding muscular movement occurs as the result of acetylcholine release at the neuromuscular junction. Excitatory axon collaterals of the motor neuron activate (by releasing acetylcholine) an inhibitory interneuron, which fires and feedback-inhibits the motor neuron. This inhibitory effect is mediated by the release of the amino acid glycine from the axons of the inhibitory cell. Interaction between glycine and its receptors on the motor neuron increases chloride conductance into the motor neuron, which antagonizes excitatory events. When a new stimulus arrives (a local depolarization due to sodium influx), the impulse tends to die out unless it is so strong that it overcomes the inhibition.

37

The crucial role of inhibition in preserving normal neuronal function can be readily demonstrated in the living animal by administering the glycine receptor antagonist strychnine. By blocking the receptor through which glycine mediates spinal motor neuron recurrent inhibition, strychnine allows repetitive muscle movements to occur in response to single excitatory afferent input. Since the input to these motor neurons is primarily of sensory origin, loud noise or tactile stimulation causes a strychnine convulsion, ie, an exaggerated reflex response to a given afferent stimulus. Analogous excitation-inhibition mechanisms operate in most neuronal systems in the brain, although the main inhibitory transmitter in the brain is GABA, rather than glycine.

It can readily be seen that a drug can modify the normal state of neuronal function by any of a number of mechanisms. A drug can mimic or block the effect of an endogenous transmitter by causing or preventing a change in a neuronal membrane's ionic conductance. A drug can interfere with the neuronal reuptake mechanism or enzymatic catabolism that terminates the action of a neurotransmitter. For example, the tricyclic antidepressants block the reuptake of the monoamine neurotransmitters, and monoamine oxidase inhibitors (antihypertensive and antidepressant drugs) decrease the rate of monoamine catabolism. Both effects result in more transmitter being made available to interact with its receptors per unit time. Virtually all centrally active drugs, including sedatives, hypnotics, and analgesics, are believed to produce their effects either by acting as receptor agonists, by affecting transmitter-receptor interactions, or by altering membrane ionic conductances via a direct interaction with the membrane.

BENZODIAZEPINES

Unlike the barbiturates, benzodiazepines do not produce marked respiratory depression; therefore, they are far safer than the barbiturates and have largely replaced them as sedatives and hypnotics. Also unlike the barbiturates, benzodiazepines are not general depressants of neuronal activity. They are similar to other classes of drugs that decrease CNS activity, however, in that they produce a variety of effects, depending on dose. In addition to being widely used as sedatives and hypnotics, benzodiazepines are effective muscle relaxants and anticonvulsants. At high doses, these compounds cause a sometimes useful quasi-anesthetic state that interferes with recent memory.

The effects of benzodiazepines on the stages of sleep are relevant to their use as hypnotics. Stage 0 refers to the awake state. Stages 1 and 2 are the two stages from which the normal individual can be easily aroused, but in which the early EEG changes are observed. Stages 3 and 4 comprise deep sleep or slow-wave sleep. Rapid eye movement (REM) sleep, which is characterized by bursts of eye movements, is a stage of deep sleep in which most dreaming occurs. Benzodiazepines decrease sleep latency (the time it takes to begin sleeping), and increase the amount of time spent in stage 2, the predominant stage of non-REM sleep. The time spent in slow-wave sleep (stages 3 and 4) is also reduced. Time in REM sleep is usually shortened, but these effects seem to vary, depending on the drug and the individual. The net result of benzodiazepine treatment is an increase in total sleep time and a sense of deep, refreshing sleep. Chronic use of benzodiazepines can result in tolerance to their sleep-producing effects. Withdrawal can result in REM rebound, ie, an increase in dreaming and a decrease in total sleep time.

This class of drugs includes diazepam, chlordiazepoxide, flunitrazepam, flurazepam, nitrazepam, oxazepam, prazepam, triazolam, and others. Benzodiazepines are used as follows:

1. Hypnotic in treatment of insomnia
2. Sedative in treatment of anxiety
3. Muscle relaxant in spastic states
4. Anticonvulsant in treatment of status epilepticus
5. Adjunctive therapy for preanesthesia and anesthesia

Mechanism of Action

Benzodiazepines are believed to act by potentiating GABA-mediated neuronal inhibition. This potentiation is thought to depend on the presence of GABA itself, not on a GABA receptor agonist action. They do not bind to the GABA receptor site in vitro. Accordingly, depletion of GABA antagonizes the effects of benzodiazepines. The exact mechanism by which these compounds potentiate GABA-mediated effects is unknown, but it could involve an action on the GABA receptor at other than the active site to facilitate the conformational change produced by GABA. Recent evidence suggests that benzodiazepines may act on a protein called GABA-modulin, which normally down-regulates the GABA receptor. Benzodiazepines may cause GABA-modulin to be phosphorylated, and thereby inactivated, resulting in a decrease in GABA receptor down-regulation. Regardless of the exact way in which benzodiazepines potentiate GABA's effects, the increase in GABA receptor activation increases the GABA-mediated inhibition of cells, thereby decreasing neuronal activity and reducing the response of neurons to excitatory input. The involvement of GABA-mediated inhibition in many neuronal systems is probably the reason that benzodiazepines have a multitude of useful effects. The actual sites within the brain where these compounds act to produce their pharmacologic effects are unknown, however.

Pharmacokinetics

Benzodiazepines are absorbed from the gastrointestinal (GI) tract and some (eg, diazepam) are highly bound by plasma proteins. Diazepam, nitrazepam, and others undergo enterohepatic circulation after hepatic metabolism. The fact that elimination half-lives vary can be used to advantage. For example, because the rate of elimination of benzodiazepines is slower in the elderly than in younger persons, a benzodiazepine with a relatively short half-life (eg, oxazepam) may be preferable for an elderly patient in order to avoid CNS depression in the morning.

Adverse Effects

Benzodiazepines are generally well tolerated, but dependence can develop with chronic use or abuse. Acute effects include confusion, dysarthria, motor incoordination, CNS depression, retrograde amnesia, and dry mouth. In addition, tolerance may develop with chronic use, and this is a reason for cessation of therapy. Abrupt cessation can result in a withdrawal syndrome featuring rebound insomnia, anxiety, agitation, and depression. Cessation of chronic therapy with benzodiazepines possessing anticonvulsant activity, eg, diazepam, can precipitate withdrawal convulsions.

BARBITURATES

Considered general depressants of excitable tissue, barbiturates have many effects on many tissues. At clinically used doses, however, the CNS is the primary site of barbiturate action. Barbiturates at various doses produce all degrees of CNS depression, and this property is the main drawback to the use of barbiturates. Although effective to induce sleep, barbiturates produce respiratory depression at higher doses and have therefore been widely and successfully used for suicide.

As sedatives and hypnotics, the barbiturates have been largely superseded by the benzodiazepines. Barbiturates are still useful in anesthesia (eg, thiopental and pentobarbital) and in the treatment of chronic epilepsy (eg, phenobarbital). Currently used barbiturates include amobarbital, hexobarbital, pentobarbital, phenobarbital, and secobarbital. They are used for

1. Sedation (superseded by benzodiazepines)
2. Hypnosis (superseded by benzodiazepines)
3. Epilepsy (phenobarbital used chronically in treatment of seizure disorders)
4. Intravenous anesthesia
5. Status epilepticus (superseded by benzodiazepines)
6. Induction of neonatal hepatic metabolism in jaundice

Mechanism of Action

The available evidence suggests that barbiturates act to potentiate GABA-mediated inhibition, although the mechanism by which they do so is unclear. Even though a GABA-related mechanism may underlie the pharmacologic actions of both the barbiturates and the benzodiazepines, there are important differences between these two classes of drugs. The therapeutic index for barbiturates is much lower than the index for benzodiazepines, since barbiturates are general inhibitors of excitable tissue. This action of barbiturates results in significant respiratory depression, with clinical doses higher than those used for hypnosis and sedation.

Pharmacokinetics

Barbiturates are readily absorbed from the GI tract. Plasma protein binding varies among barbiturates and is proportional to the lipid solubility of each drug. Weak acids, such as aspirin and warfarin, can displace barbiturates from plasma protein binding sites. Highly lipid-soluble barbiturates, eg, thiopental, distribute quickly into the rapidly perfused tissues of the body. This results in a short-latency, short-duration anesthesia as the drug redistributes into the body fat and other tissues.

Barbiturates are filtered by the kidney, but most of the lipid-soluble barbiturates are reabsorbed passively. Those barbiturates that are weak acids, eg, phenobarbital, are excreted in the urine. Osmotic diuresis and alkalinization of the urine increase the rate of phenobarbital excretion. Those drugs not excreted in the urine are metabolized by the liver and other tissues. As mentioned previously, a barbiturate's half-life is affected by prior exposure to the drug, since barbiturates are capable of inducing microsomal drug metabolism. Half-lives are increased in pregnant patients because of an increase in plasma protein binding and in patients with hepatic disease because of decreased drug metabolism.

Adverse Effects

Undesired drowsiness, diffuse pain, and paradoxical excitement may result from the administration of barbiturates. A preferential depression of inhibitory mechanisms may lead to the excitatory effect. Barbiturates can also depress the excitable tissue of the heart so that rapid intravenous injection can cause cardiovenous collapse before respiratory depression occurs. Barbiturates are absolutely contraindicated in porphyria, since these compounds increase porphyrin synthesis.

3
Analgesics

Pain can be divided into two components. One is the actual physical sensation mediated by sensory neuronal pathways; the other is the reaction to the stimulus, ie, the emotional response that amplifies pain. The first component involves neurophysiological mechanisms that are at least partially understood, and it is on these that analgesics are believed to act. The recent discovery of endogenous opioid peptides has shed considerable light on opiate analgesics' mechanisms of action and their relationship to pain mechanisms.

It is well-known that a variety of tissues respond biologically to morphine. The CNS responds to morphine with analgesia, euphoria, tolerance, addiction, and respiratory depression. The contractile activity of the vas deferens and the gut is decreased by morphine. The awareness that morphine receptors mediate the pharmacologic effects of morphine long preceded the demonstration of in vitro morphine binding to tissue homogenates. However, it was Hughes, Kosterlitz, and colleagues who found in 1975 that an extract of mammalian brain decreases the contractions of vas deferens much as morphine does and that the opiate antagonist naloxone blocks this brain extract–induced relaxation of vas deferens. They then isolated, identified, and synthesized the active compounds and showed that the synthetic pentapeptides produce a morphinelike effect that is blocked by naloxone. These two compounds are methionine- and leucine-enkephalin. Subsequent intensive investigation has shown that there are many different opioid peptide receptors and that many endogenous peptides, such as β-endorphin, dynorphin, the enkephalins, and a bewildering variety of other newly discovered peptides, act at these peptide receptors.

According to one current view, afferent input to the spinal cord from sensory pathways evokes spinal neuron activity that is relayed to the brain and perceived as pain. It has been postulated that interneurons, using endogenous opioid peptides as neurotransmitters, innervate the incoming sensory nerve terminals and decrease the release of excitatory transmitter (possibly Substance P). According to this view, morphine is an exogenous ligand for the endogenous opioid peptide receptor and mimics the effect of the endogenous opioid peptide transmitter, thereby decreasing the afferent (painful) stimulus. Although any theory may ultimately be shown to be invalid or only partially correct, this hypothesis is at least a useful way in which to view the interaction between exogenous analgesics and endogenous pain mechanisms.

NARCOTIC ANALGESICS

Morphine and its many semisynthetic congeners are considered narcotic analgesics. Morphine exerts profound effects primarily on two organs, the CNS and the gut. Centrally, morphine produces analgesia without loss of consciousness, drowsiness, or changes in mood. Other centrally mediated effects include pupillary constriction and respiratory depression. Morphine and its congeners are markedly different from other classes of centrally acting drugs. Barbiturates, alcohol, and inhalation anesthetics all produce analgesia, for example, but they also produce ataxia leading to unconsciousness, slurred speech, and other signs of CNS depression. At effective analgesic doses, morphine does not cause these effects; furthermore, mental clouding is markedly less with morphine than with other drugs. Morphine does, however, produce nausea and vomiting. The position of the individual determines whether these effects occur. Because patients in the standing position are more sensitive to morphine's emetic effects, a vestibular involvement is assumed. Another major property of morphine used clinically before morphine was given as an analgesic, is its inhibitory effect on gut motility; it slows the rate of digestion and passage of the intestinal contents, resulting in constipation. Morphine also decreases uterine contractility and antagonizes oxytocics.

The other major class of narcotic analgesics includes meperidine and its congeners. Meperidine has analgesic actions similar to those of morphine and acts by the same mechanism, but it is not useful as an antitussive or antidiarrheal. Meperidine has negligible effects on uterine activity and is not antioxytocic. Both morphine and meperidine cross the placenta. Therefore, the neonate of a mother who was given one of these drugs in labor may exhibit respiratory depression. Meperidine produces less respiratory depression in the neonate than does morphine.

Narcotic analgesics have the following uses:

1. Analgesia: morphine, codeine, meperidine, oxycodone, hydrocodone, hydromorphone, oxymorphone, pentazocine, propoxyphene
2. Diarrhea: opium tincture, diphenoxylate, loperamide
3. Antitussive: codeine, dextromethorphan, levopropoxyphene, noscapine
4. Dyspnea, particularly dyspnea of acute left ventricular failure and pulmonary edema: morphine
5. Preanesthesia and anesthesia: morphine, fentanyl

Mechanism of Action

The discovery of the endogenous opioid peptides leucine-enkephalin, methi-onine-enkephalin, β-endorphin, dynorphin, and others has elucidated to a considerable degree the mechanism of exogenous opiates' action. These endogenous peptides are thought to be neurotransmitters or neuromodulators in the CNS. Accordingly, morphine and its congeners are believed to act as exogenous opioid peptide receptor agonists that mimic the effects of the endogenous peptides. Since there are different peptides in different cells in many parts of the CNS, the many central effects of morphine may be the result of its simultaneous effects on opioid peptide receptors that mediate different functions. Although intensive study is currently under way to determine the precise sites of action of morphine's effects, a considerable amount of information already is available.

ANALGESIA

The analgesic effects of morphine are believed to be partly due to an action in the spinal cord. According to this view, endogenous opioid peptides and exogenous opiates decrease transmitter release from the afferent fibers that initiate the pain process by exciting spinal neurons. The endogenous peptides appear to be localized in spinal interneurons, and it is hypothesized that endogenous opioid peptides are released onto the presynaptic terminals of afferent pain fibers, thereby decreasing transmitter release. It is thought that exogenous opiates, eg, morphine, interact with the same receptor to reduce activity in the pathway and, thus, reduce pain. The mechanisms underlying the other central effects of opiates, such as mood changes and mental clouding, remain to be elucidated. It has been found that periventricular and periaqueductal regions may also be sites of action for morphine's analgesic effects. These areas bind opiates avidly. Interestingly, the amygdala, a brain region rich in opiate binding sites, does not appear to be involved in morphine analgesia, which suggests that some of morphine's other central effects may involve amygdalar mechanisms. This, however, remains a subject of conjecture.

With chronic administration of any opiate or opiatelike drug, the dose must be increased to produce the same pharmacologic effect (tolerance). Although some of the reduced response to a given dose may be due to an increase in the rate of drug metabolism, tolerance is characterized by a change in the neuronal response to the presence of the drug. The nature of this neuronal response is unknown. It has been suggested that opioid drugs inhibit an enzyme (possibly adenyl cyclase) or enzymatic process that mediates the effects of opiates. According to this view, enzyme inhibition results in a decreased rate of product formation (possibly cAMP). This decrease in product, in turn, leads to feedback stimulation of enzyme synthesis. Increased enzyme synthesis requires more drug to produce the same level of enzyme inhibition, thus explaining tolerance. This model also provides an explanation for withdrawal phenomena. Removal of opiate drugs from an opiate-tolerant person allows the supranormal amount of now uninhibited enzyme to produce its product in abnormally large amounts. It is implied in this model that the cellular processes stimulated by the enzymatic product mediate the withdrawal signs, ie, lacrimation, sweating, runny nose, dilated pupils, anorexia, irritability, tremor, insomnia, sneezing, depression, nausea, vomiting, and diarrhea, as well as widespread muscle cramping and an overwhelming feeling of misery. This unpleasant withdrawal syndrome develops spontaneously within 2 to 3 days after the last dose of an opiate drug or can be precipitated abruptly in dependent individuals by injection of an opiate receptor antagonist, eg, naloxone. The physiological signs of the syndrome are believed to result from the rebound facilitation of CNS processes that have been depressed in the tolerant state, and blockade of the opiate receptors pharmacologically with naloxone releases these processes, causing an immediate withdrawal syndrome.

PUPILLARY CONSTRICTION

A ubiquitous feature of opiate use is pupillary constriction. This appears to be due to an action on the oculomotor nerve rather than to a direct action on the eye. Pupillary constriction can be reversed by injection of the opiate receptor antagonist naloxone. Therefore, naloxone is used to determine if an individual is using opiates as well as to treat opiate overdose.

RESPIRATORY DEPRESSION

A major central effect of morphine, one that limits its usefulness therapeutically, is respiratory depression. Morphine probably produces respiratory depression by reducing brain stem response to increased P_{CO_2}. Morphine also inhibits respiratory rhythmicity by actions in pontine and medullary centers; these effects are presumably mediated by opioid peptide receptors.

COUGH REFLEX AND EMESIS

Morphine suppresses the cough reflex and causes emesis by direct actions in the brain stem, also presumably mediated by opioid peptide receptor activation.

GASTROINTESTINAL EFFECTS

Morphine acts at various sites of the gastrointestinal (GI) tract to decrease intestinal activity and the rate of passage of intestinal contents. It acts on the duodenum to decrease the rate at which stomach contents pass into the small intestine. Propulsive movements of the small and large intestine are decreased, and the tone of the ileocecal valve and the anal sphincter is increased. It has also been suggested that the central effects of morphine blunt the centrally mediated response to colonic fullness. Morphine's direct actions on the bowel presumably are mediated by opioid peptide receptors, and these actions can be blocked by naloxone.

The physiological role of endogenous opioid peptides in the intestine remains unclear, so the exact mechanism by which morphine decreases intestinal activity is unknown. Some evidence suggests that opiate receptor stimulation decreases acetylcholine release in the guinea pig ileum; thus, opioid peptides may decrease presynaptic transmitter release, thereby decreasing any neuronally mediated effect in which they are involved. In addition to its direct effects on the gut, morphine decreases gut activity by central mechanisms. Injection of morphine directly into the brain decreases gut activity, and this effect can be blocked by opiate receptor antagonists or by vagotomy. Therefore, a central inhibition of vagal output by morphine is likely.

Pharmacokinetics

MORPHINE, CODEINE, AND HEROIN

Morphine is readily absorbed from all routes of administration, but, because of a significant first-pass effect, the plasma concentration after oral administration is lower than that after parenteral administration. The main route of metabolism of morphine is glucuronidation. Codeine and its derivatives possess a methoxy group in the 3 position, and this partially prevents the first-pass effect. Therefore, codeine is relatively effective when taken orally. A portion of the codeine administered is demethylated to form morphine, however, and it is this morphine that is responsible for codeine's analgesic effects. Similarly, heroin (diacetylmorphine) is deacetylated in the brain to morphine. The "rush" obtained after heroin injection is apparently due to the rapid entry of this more lipid-soluble version of morphine into the brain and the resulting high brain concentrations of morphine after deacetylation. Therefore, both heroin and codeine can be considered slightly modified morphine molecules that are subsequently converted by the body to the active molecule, morphine.

Approximately one third of circulating morphine is bound to plasma proteins. The half-life of morphine in young adults is 2.5 to 3 hours. Morphine distributes widely, and the major route of elimination of morphine and its glucuronide is the kidney. Enterohepatic circulation of morphine-glucuronide occurs.

MEPERIDINE AND CONGENERS

Meperidine, like morphine, is readily absorbed by all routes of administration. Approximately 60% of circulating meperidine is bound to plasma proteins. It is metabolized primarily by the liver, and, after oral administration, only half the administered dose survives the first pass through the liver. Meperidine is metabolized by hydrolysis, conjugation, and N-demethylation to form normeperidine.

With the administration of toxic doses, the normeperidine accumulates. Unlike meperidine, normeperidine is an excitant; therefore, meperidine overdose can cause a mixture of CNS depression (due to meperidine) and convulsions (due to normeperidine). This syndrome has been seen in patients with renal failure, since normeperidine concentrations increase when renal excretion is impaired. A recent study in cancer patients has also shown that normeperidine-induced excitation (tremors, twitches, myoclonus, and seizures) may occur in the absence of renal impairment.

Adverse Effects

The majority of adverse effects of morphine and other opiates are related to their actions on opioid peptide receptors. Such effects include mental clouding, respiratory depression, constipation, nausea, and vomiting. Constipation and vomiting are less common with meperidine. Pentazocine often causes hallucinogenic effects that can be blocked by naloxone, suggesting that this effect is due to an opioid peptide receptor agonist action.

NONNARCOTIC ANALGESICS

Aspirin (acetylsalicylic acid) and related salicylates (eg, sodium salicylate, methyl salicylate, and salicylic acid), as well as acetaminophen and phenacetin, are nonnarcotic analgesics. Used for pain of low to moderate intensity, they are more effective for the treatment of dull pain arising from inflammatory processes than they are for sharp, stabbing pain of any origin. The maximal analgesic efficacy of this class of drugs is far less than that of the opiate analgesics (with the possible exception of propoxyphene), but the aspirinlike drugs may be just as effective as the opiate analgesics for low to moderate pain associated with inflammatory conditions. Furthermore, this class of analgesics does not produce tolerance, addiction, or marked respiratory depression, nor do they block other sensations as do the opiates. All drugs of this class possess antiinflammatory, antipyretic, and analgesic activity, but acetaminophen is markedly less antiinflammatory than are the others of the group.

It is impossible to separate the analgesic actions of this class of compounds from their antipyretic and antiinflammatory effects, since their common mechanism of action (inhibition of prostaglandin synthesis) affects all three processes. Some drugs of this class are used primarily for their antiinflammatory activity, eg, phenylbutazone, naproxen, fenoprofen, diflunisal, ibuprofen, indomethacin, sulindac, and tolmetin. These drugs are closely related to the aspirinlike analgesics in terms of their mechanism of action and pharmacologic properties, however, and they may be promoted in the future for analgesia as well as for arthritis.

Since this class of compounds is believed to act by inhibiting prostaglandin, prostacyclin, and thromboxane synthesis, all drugs of the class affect virtually any physiological or pathologic process mediated by these endogenous compounds. For example, because platelet aggregation involves thromboxane A_2, aspirin and related drugs inhibit platelet aggregation and prolong bleeding time. Aspirin relieves some of the signs and symptoms of dysmenorrhea, since prostaglandins apparently play a role in the uterine contractions that occur during menstruation. Aspirin also prolongs gestation by inhibiting the synthesis of prostaglandins that play a role in uterine contraction at birth. Similarly, prostaglandins are apparently involved in maintaining a patent ductus arteriosis, and aspirinlike drugs have been used successfully to treat this condition. In summary, these compounds are used for

1. Analgesia
2. Inflammatory processes
3. Fever
4. Closure of a patent ductus arteriosis
5. Antiaggregant, eg, in coronary artery disease or myocardial infarction

It seems likely that continued elucidation of the role of prostaglandins in normal and diseased states will suggest new, additional uses for this class of drugs. The global role of the many metabolites of arachidonic acid in a variety of physiological processes makes the indiscriminate use of this class of drugs inadvisable, however. Attempts to produce selective changes in processes mediated by particular prostacyclins, leukotrienes, and prostaglandins will await the development of new, more selective compounds.

Mechanism of Action

As discussed previously, the salicylates and salicylatelike analgesics, eg, aspirin, acetaminophen, and phenacetin, are believed to produce their main pharmacologic effects by inhibiting the synthesis and release of prostaglandins and other products of arachidonic acid. In order to understand how these drugs work, it is necessary to understand the mammalian metabolism of arachidonic acid, the precursor of prostaglandins, prostacyclins, thromboxanes, and leukotrienes. Arachidonic acid, ingested as a constituent of meat or produced in vivo from dietary linoleic acid, is attached to membrane phospholipids. Phospholipase A_2 liberates arachidonic acid from the membrane, which may be the rate-limiting step for its metabolism.

Free arachidonic acid is metabolized by two enzymes, lipoxygenase and cyclooxygenase. Lipoxygenase converts arachidonic acid into a class of compounds called leukotrienes, which are noncyclized, 20-carbon carboxylic acids. These leukotrienes apparently play an as yet undetermined role in inflammatory processes. Much more is known about the products of cyclooxygenase. Arachidonic acid is converted to prostaglandin G_2 (PGG_2) and then to prostaglandin H_2 (PGH_2) by cyclooxygenase. PGH_2 is converted to PGE_2, $PGF_{2\alpha}$, and prostaglandin D_2 (PGD_2). PGH_2 is also converted to thromboxane A_2 (TXA_2) via thromboxane synthetase and then to the stable thromboxane B_2 (TXB_2). In addition, PGH_2 can be metabolized to prostacyclin (PGI_2) via prostacyclin synthetase.

A number of major points about the products of cyclooxygenase action are now clear. First, all cells studied have the microsomal enzymes necessary to produce prostaglandins. Second, prostaglandins are not stored, but are synthesized and released when the cells are stimulated to do so; this always occurs when cells are damaged. Third, aspirin and all related drugs inhibit the synthesis and release of prostaglandins. Because they inhibit the first cyclooxygenase step, they decrease the production of all prostaglandins, thromboxanes, and prostacyclins. Different drugs of this class inhibit the fatty acid cyclooxygenase by different mechanisms. Aspirin (acetylsalicylic acid) acts by acetylating a serine molecule at the active site of the enzyme. Salicylic acid, which lacks the acetyl group of aspirin, and the other drugs of this class act by other, less clear mechanisms.

Release of the products of cyclooxygenase into the blood is believed to be the cause of some types of inflammation and pain. This conclusion is supported by the observations that injections of PGE_2 or $PGF_{2\alpha}$ used to induce abortion cause severe local pain and that intravenous injection of prostaglandins causes headache and vascular pain. It remains to be elucidated whether prostaglandins directly evoke a pain sensation or produce pain by sensitizing the tissue to the pain-producing effect of a peptide, eg, bradykinin. Either way, aspirin and related drugs are believed to block only the pain mediated by the synthesis and release of prostaglandins, thromboxanes, and related metabolites of cyclooxygenase products. In contrast to the central effects of opiate drugs, these analgesic effects are peripheral in origin and do not take place in the absence of an inflammatory process.

Acetaminophen is somewhat different from other drugs of the class. It is less antiinflammatory than the others and is only a weak inhibitor of prostaglandin synthesis. It has been suggested that acetaminophen may have more efficacy at central enzymes than at peripheral ones, which may explain acetaminophen's antipyretic and analgesic effects, as well as its relative lack of antiinflammatory activity. The fact that acetaminophen has fewer GI side-effects than aspirin may be a consequence of its somewhat different mode of action.

Pharmacokinetics

SALICYLATES (ASPIRIN, SODIUM SALICYLATE, SALICYLIC ACID)

Salicylates are readily absorbed after oral ingestion, partly from the stomach, but predominantly from the small intestine. They distribute widely, and the equilibriums formed between extracellular water and other tissue and fluid compartments are determined by pH-dependent processes. Aspirin readily crosses the placenta. It is rapidly hydrolyzed to salicylate, which is then highly bound to plasma proteins, particularly albumin. Salicylate competes with a number of drugs for protein binding sites and, therefore, can decrease the binding of other ligands, such as phenytoin, thyroxin, triiodothyronine, sulfinpyrazone, penicillin, thiopental, uric acid, naproxen, and bilirubin. In addition, acetylation of albumin by aspirin can alter the binding of other drugs, such as phenylbutazone and flufenamic acid. Salicylates are metabolized primarily by the liver to a glycine conjugate and to glucuronides.

Salicylates and their conjugates are excreted primarily by the kidney. Although the pH of the urine does not affect the excretion rate of salicylate conjugates, the excretion of salicylate itself is highly dependent on urinary pH. At an acid pH, salicylate is mainly in the uncharged (protonated) form; therefore, it is reabsorbed from the glomerular filtrate into the blood. Conversely, in an alkaline urine, salicylate is predominantly in the charged (unprotonated) form, resulting in decreased reabsorption and an increased rate of excretion. The plasma half-life of aspirin is approximately 15 minutes. The half-life for salicylate is 2 to 3 hours with low doses, but 15 to 30 hours with high doses because of a rate-limiting step of hepatic metabolism.

ACETAMINOPHEN AND PHENACETIN

Acetaminophen is rapidly absorbed after oral ingestion and distributes widely throughout the body. Plasma protein binding is limited at therapeutic doses. Acetaminophen is metabolized by the liver to a variety of conjugates, which are excreted in the urine. Phenacetin is the precursor of acetaminophen, and most of an administered dose of phenacetin is rapidly converted by the liver to acetaminophen. Phenacetin is also metabolized by the liver to a large number of other compounds. The acetaminophen plasma half-life is 1 to 3 hours.

Adverse Effects

All nonnarcotic analgesics share some adverse effects related to decreased prostaglandin synthesis, since they have this mechanism of action in common. As mentioned earlier, prostaglandin synthesis inhibitors prolong bleeding time and gestation. In addition, the use of salicylates prior to and during delivery can increase postpartum bleeding, as well as perinatal mortality, anemia, and complications in delivery. Another adverse effect of many of these drugs is GI bleeding. The cause of GI bleeding is not clear, but it may be due partly to inhibition of the normal role of prostaglandins in gastric blood flow, mucous secretion, and platelet aggregation.

Acetaminophen in overdosage may have a fatal hepatotoxic effect. Ingestion of more than 6 g acetaminophen can increase the rate of the first step of acetaminophen metabolism to such a degree that the glutathione needed to convert the product of this first step to harmless metabolites is depleted. A toxic intermediate (probably N-acetyl-p-benzoquinone) accumulates and binds to liver cell constituents, causing a potentially fatal hepatic necrosis. Although the main active metabolite of phenacetin is acetaminophen, phenacetin overdose does not cause this hepatotoxic reaction, apparently because the rate at which acetaminophen is formed from phenacetin never exceeds the ability of the liver to metabolize it normally. However, phenacetin can be converted to an unknown, but toxic, metabolite that causes methemoglobinemia and hemolytic anemia. This can occur in patients who ingest an overdosage of phenacetin or in patients who metabolize phenacetin preferentially to the toxic metabolite.

Although aspirin causes neither a hepatotoxic reaction nor methemoglobinemia, salicylates are often consumed in overdosage, resulting in salicylism. This condition is characterized by headache, dizziness, ringing in the ears (tinnitus), impaired vision, confusion, drowsiness, lassitude, sweating, thirst, nausea, vomiting, and hyperventilation.

4

Drugs Used in Cardiovascular and Hypertensive Diseases

ANTIHYPERTENSIVE DRUGS

The drugs that are useful in the treatment of elevated blood pressure, whether of known or unknown causes, can be divided into six categories:

1. Drugs that decrease blood pressure by a centrally mediated action that decreases sympathetic nervous system activity, eg, methyldopa and clonidine

2. Drugs that act directly on the postganglionic sympathetic nerves to decrease sympathetic tone to the heart and vascular smooth muscle, eg, guanethidine, reserpine, and monoamine oxidase inhibitors

3. Drugs that circumvent the sympathetic nervous system and act directly on the adrenergic receptors innervated by the sympathetic nerves, eg, phentolamine, prazosin, and propranolol

4. Drugs that bypass both the sympathetic nerves and their postsynaptic adrenergic receptors and act to relax vascular smooth muscle directly, eg, hydralazine, diazoxide, and nitroprusside

5. Drugs that act on the kidney to increase sodium and therefore water excretion, eg, the thiazide diuretics

6. Drugs that antagonize the renin-angiotensin system that normally maintains and increases vascular tone, eg, captopril

The sympathetic and parasympathetic innervations of peripheral target organs are disynaptic. That is, two cells constitute each pathway from brain stem or spinal cord to the effector site. The cell bodies of the first cells of sympathetic nerves lie in the spinal cord, but their terminals usually reside in ganglia outside the spinal cord in a paravertebral chain or elsewhere. These cells use acetylcholine as a transmitter in the ganglia. The axons of these cells are called preganglionic fibers. The first cell of the parasympathetic nerves terminates closer to the effector organ, often within its tissue. These preganglionic parasympathetic fibers also utilize acetylcholine as a transmitter. Therefore, *all preganglionic fibers, whether sympathetic or parasympathetic, use acetylcholine as a transmitter.* They release acetylcholine to the postganglionic cells that possess cholinergic receptors and acetylcholinesterase needed to metabolize the released acetylcholine. The postganglionic parasympathetic nerves that innervate so many peripheral organs also use acetylcholine as a transmitter. Only the postganglionic sympathetic fibers use norepinephrine as a transmitter.

One interesting variant involves the adrenal medulla. The preganglionic, sympathetic, cholinergic fibers innervate the adrenal medulla and, when activated, cause the adrenal medullary cells to release norepinephrine and epinephrine directly into the blood. Therefore, the adrenal medullary cells can be regarded as a specialized collection of postganglionic sympathetic cells that "innervate" the blood, rather than an organ. The blood receives the released catecholamines in order to transport them to the ultimate destination, eg, the heart.

The primary purpose of the autonomic nervous system is regulation. Many organs under autonomic control have an intrinsic level of activity even after denervation; eg, the heart will pump and the intestinal smooth muscle will contract after removal of parasympathetic and sympathetic innervation. Most organs are innervated by both sympathetic and parasympathetic nerves. These two inputs often have opposing actions to provide a means of up- and down-regulation from an organ's basal level of activity. For example, when activated, the parasympathetic input to the heart depresses cardiac activity, and the sympathetic input increases heart rate and contractility. This is not a general rule, however, since some targets of autonomic activity, such as the sweat glands, do not have a basal level of activity and need only one control to activate them.

As stated earlier, all preganglionic fibers, whether sympathetic or parasympathetic, use acetylcholine as a transmitter. So do the postganglionic parasympathetic fibers. In addition, the nonautonomic motor nerves originating in the spinal cord and innervating skeletal muscle use acetylcholine as a transmitter. Although these three pathways use the same transmitter, the postsynaptic receptors for acetylcholine are different. Therefore, different cholinergic drugs have different pharmacologic effects and side-effects, depending on their affinity for each type of cholinergic receptor. There are two main types of acetylcholine receptor, which were originally discriminated on the basis of their reactions to the application of muscarine and nicotine. Because the ganglionic acetylcholine receptors and the acetylcholine receptors at the neuromuscular junction are activated by nicotine, they are termed nicotinic receptors. These nicotinic receptors are not identical, however, and react differently to different nicotinic agonists and antagonists. The other type of acetylcholine receptor, termed muscarinic, is the receptor type that mediates all postganglionic parasympathetic effects.

Since parasympathetic fibers innervate the heart, lungs, salivary and lacrimal glands, pupil, gastrointestinal (GI) tract, and bladder, injection of a muscarinic cholinergic agonist, eg, methacholine, produces a variety of cholinergic effects concomitantly. The prominent signs of muscarinic cholinergic excess are salivation, lacrimation, urination, and diarrhea (SLUD). The muscarinic cholinergic receptor antagonist atropine blocks these effects of the agonist methacholine by competitive inhibition at all muscarinic cholinergic receptors.

The sympathetic branch of the autonomic nervous system also utilizes different receptors in different tissues. All postganglionic sympathetic nerve fibers release norepinephrine; the adrenal medulla releases both norepinephrine and epinephrine. The sympathetic nerves play a central role in mammals' "fight-or-flight" reaction. When escape or defense mechanisms are needed, there is a general burst of sympathetic activity to increase respiration, metabolic energy, and blood flow to the heart and skeletal muscles. In order to maximize efficiency, blood flow through nonessential tissues, such as the GI tract, skin, and fat, must be decreased. The need to open some blood vessels, eg, coronary and skeletal muscle arteries, and to close others, eg, mesenteric and skin vessels, led to the evolutionary development of the α-adrenergic and β-adrenergic receptors. Although all sympathetic fibers release the same chemical, ie, norepinephrine, responses vary because cell membranes possess different receptors that bind the same ligand, but mediate different biologic effects. Sympathetic discharge increases blood flow to heart muscle via β-adrenergic receptors in coronary artery smooth muscle and increases heart rate and contractility via β-adrenergic receptors in the cardiac conduction system and in the heart muscle itself. Blood flow to skeletal muscle increases, and bronchial muscles relax via β-adrenergic receptors that mediate smooth muscle relaxation. Conversely, sympathetic discharge causes vasoconstriction to reduce blood flow in the GI tract, skin, and fat via α-adrenergic receptors that mediate vasoconstriction. It was recently discovered that there are two subsets of β-adrenergic receptors, termed β_1 and β_2. The slight differences in three-dimensional configuration between the two receptor types led to the development of drugs that have more or less affinity for one or the other β-adrenergic receptors. The β-adrenergic receptors in the heart muscle and conduction system are of the β_1 type; those in the arterioles of the heart, skeletal muscle, lung, kidney, gut, and uterus are of the β_2 type. Clinically, these differences between β_1- and β_2-adrenergic receptors are exploited in the treatment of asthma. An asthmatic individual can obtain relief by inhaling epinephrine, an endogenous β-adrenergic receptor agonist. But epinephrine not only relaxes bronchial muscle to improve breathing (a β_2 action), but also stimulates the heart (a β_1 action). Cardiac stimulation is undesirable in some patients, so terbutaline, a drug with greater affinity for the β_2-adrenergic receptor, was developed to treat asthma without causing marked cardiac effects.

Recent experimental evidence has suggested that there are also subtypes of α-adrenergic receptors. The α_1-adrenergic receptor is the traditional postsynaptic α-adrenergic receptor, and the α_2-adrenergic receptor is postulated to be a presynaptic receptor that, when activated, inhibits transmitter release. The existence and functional significance of α_2-adrenergic receptors are subjects of current conjecture and controversy.

Centrally Acting Antihypertensives

METHYLDOPA

Blood pressure and total peripheral resistance decrease when methyldopa is given. Unlike drugs that act directly on postganglionic sympathetic nerves to deplete norepinephrine, eg, guanethidine and reserpine, methyldopa therapy does not abolish sympathetic reflexes. Therefore, it does not produce postural hypotension as commonly as does guanethidine or reserpine. Methyldopa decreases renin secretion slightly, but this effect is not believed to play a significant role in its antihypertensive effect. Methyldopa is useful primarily for the treatment of essential hypertension, and it is usually given in combination with a thiazide diuretic.

Mechanism of Action. Methyldopa is structurally similar to norepinephrine and its precursor levodopa. Therefore, it is subjected to a number of metabolic conversions normally intended for endogenous compounds. It is now thought that the antihypertensive effects of methyldopa are due to the direct α-adrenergic receptor agonist action of α-methylnorepinephrine. It was originally found that methyldopa was an inhibitor of l-aromatic amino acid decarboxylase (dopa decarboxylase); therefore, it was suggested that methyldopa might act to deplete peripheral norepinephrine by inhibiting its synthesis. Next, it was suggested that methyldopa might be converted in peripheral nerve to α-methylnorepinephrine, which might then be released as a "false transmitter" without receptor affinity, thereby causing a decreased sympathetic effect. Although α-methylnorepinephrine is produced in peripheral nerve, it is an effective α-adrenergic receptor ligand and causes a sympathomimetic, rather than a sympatholytic effect. Recent evidence has led to the conclusion that methyldopa crosses the blood-brain barrier and undergoes conversion to α-methylnorepinephrine which, when released, produces a central α-adrenergic receptor–mediated decrease in sympathetic activity. This competitive, central inhibition of sympathetic activity is consistent with the observation that sympathetic reflexes are not abolished by methyldopa as they are by drugs that deplete the peripheral stores of norepinephrine, eg, guanethidine and reserpine.

Pharmacokinetics. Methyldopa is erratically absorbed from the GI tract. Much of an orally administered dose is metabolized, suggesting a first-pass effect by the liver. The decrease in blood pressure is maximal 4 to 6 hours after oral administration, and the plasma half-life is approximately 2 hours. The antihypertensive effects are evident up to 24 hours after an oral dose, probably because neuronal methyldopa and metabolites are stored presynaptically and remain long after the plasma concentrations fall. Methyldopa is excreted mainly via the kidneys, but renal impairment is not a main determinant in consideration of the dose.

Adverse Effects. Methyldopa often causes marked sedation. Postural hypotension due to central inhibition of sympathetic function can occur, but it is more likely to occur after the administration of guanethidine or reserpine. Similarly, ejaculatory failure is less common with methyldopa than with guanethidine or reserpine (ejaculation is a sympathetically mediated reflex) since methyldopa leaves sympathetic reflexes intact. Dry mouth, nasal stuffiness, vertigo, extrapyramidal effects, lactation, and depression of mood are also seen; these are most likely additional central effects of methyldopa or its active metabolites. Adverse effects probably unrelated to methyldopa's central action include fever with shaking chills, hepatic injury that can lead to necrosis, and a positive direct Coombs' test.

CLONIDINE

Like methyldopa, clonidine reduces blood pressure by a central α-adrenergic receptor–mediated mechanism. Unlike methyldopa, clonidine's effects are due to clonidine itself rather than to an active metabolite of the parent drug. After intravenous (IV) injection, there is an initial pressor response, because of a peripheral α-adrenergic receptor–mediated vasoconstriction, followed by the centrally mediated decrease in sympathetic output. Clonidine does not abolish sympathetic reflexes; the sympathetic response to exercise or the Valsalva maneuver is intact, as is the reflex control of capacitance vessels. Postural hypotension can occur but this is less common with drugs that do not abolish sympathetic reflexes than with those that do. Clonidine relaxes the renal vasculature, thus maintaining renal blood flow, and decreases plasma renin moderately.

Clonidine, usually in combination with a diuretic, is useful for the treatment of essential hypertension and may be useful in the treatment of migraine. Rebound hypertensive crisis can occur after abrupt withdrawal of clonidine. The high incidence of side-effects and the possibility of a potentially dangerous hypertensive crisis upon withdrawal limit routine use of clonidine as a first-line drug for the treatment of moderate hypertension.

Mechanism of Action and Pharmacokinetics. Clonidine, like methyldopa, is believed to be an agonist at central α-adrenergic receptors that, when activated, reduce sympathetic activity. It is absorbed from the GI tract (approximately 75% bioavailability) and largely excreted by the kidney. The half-life of the drug in the body is approximately 8 hours.

Adverse Effects. Common and severe adverse effects of clonidine therapy include the signs of central sympathetic inhibition, eg, sedation and dry mouth. Less often seen are impotence and orthostatic hypotension, also the effects of decreased sympathetic function. A hypertensive crisis upon abrupt withdrawal is to be anticipated and consists of nervousness, headache, abdominal pain, tachycardia, sweating, and hypertension that develops 8 to 12 hours after the last dose of clonidine.

Peripheral Sympatholytics

The enzymes necessary for transmitter synthesis and degradation, as well as the synaptic vesicles that store transmitter, are synthesized in the cytoplasm of the cell and transported to the sympathetic nerve endings. In the case of postganglionic sympathetic nerves, the enzymes for norepinephrine synthesis are tyrosine hydroxylase (which hydroxylates tyrosine to form dopa), l-aromatic amino acid decarboxylase (which converts dopa to dopamine), and dopamine-β-hydroxylase (which converts dopamine to norepinephrine). Norepinephrine synthesized in the vesicle from dopamine can exist free in the cytoplasm of the nerve terminal, where it is subject to degradation by the mitochondrial enzyme monoamine oxidase, or it can be stored in vesicles. When an action potential depolarizes the presynaptic terminal, norepinephrine is released into the extracellular synaptic cleft. It is unclear if transmitter release occurs from the vesicular transmitter pool, the free pool, or both. Once released, norepinephrine can

1. Interact with the postsynaptic α_1-adrenergic receptor or a postsynaptic β-adrenergic receptor,
2. Interact with a presynaptic α_2-adrenergic receptor to decrease further transmitter release (this is a subject of current controversy and disagreement),
3. Diffuse into the extracellular fluid,
4. Be degraded by the postsynaptic enzyme catechol-O-methyltransferase,
5. Be taken up by the presynaptic sympathetic terminal via the membrane uptake mechanism.

The major mechanism for transmitter inactivation is reuptake. Many of the clinically used antihypertensives produce their effects by their actions on one or more of these physiological mechanisms.

GUANETHIDINE

The initial effect of guanethidine is a transient fall in blood pressure followed by a transient increase. This is followed by a gradual fall in systemic and pulmonary blood pressure that lasts several days. The decrease in blood pressure is accompanied by bradycardia, decreased pulse pressure, and decreased cardiac output. Since guanethidine blocks sympathetic function, it decreases blood pressure most when sympathetic tone would normally be high. Therefore, guanethidine has little effect on blood pressure when the patient is in the supine position and there is normally little sympathetic tone; conversely, it greatly decreases blood pressure when the patient stands. Orthostatic hypotension and ejaculatory failure are common because sympathetic reflexes are inhibited.

Chronic use of guanethidine can result in a return of cardiac output toward normal, probably because of compensatory sodium and fluid retention, as well as increased blood volume. Plasma renin is decreased. Unlike methyldopa, clonidine, and reserpine, guanethidine does not readily pass the blood-brain barrier and, therefore, does not produce the centrally mediated effects of sedation and depression. Because guanethidine does not deplete adrenal medullary catecholamines, the physiological effects mediated by adrenal amines are not prevented by guanethidine. Guanethidine is, however, a potent drug that causes frequent and often severe adverse effects.

Guanethidine is used for moderate to severe hypertension, usually in conjunction with a diuretic, used to prevent the compensatory retention of sodium and water.

Mechanism of Action. Guanethidine has multiple effects on sympathetic nerve activity. First, it produces a bretyliumlike effect, which refers to its ability to block the release of norepinephrine from the nerve terminal. Since guanethidine possesses local anesthetic activity, this effect may be due to a local membrane action that blocks the step between depolarization and release of transmitter. This blockade of norepinephrine release in response to nerve activity occurs before the second effect of guanethidine, which is the tyraminelike effect. Guanethidine enters the synaptic vesicle and, like tyramine, releases vesicular norephinephrine into the cytoplasm, where it is subsequently metabolized by monoamine oxidase. Therefore, during chronic administration, guanethidine causes a depletion of peripheral norepinephrine stores; this effect does not occur in the adrenal medulla nor in the brain. Third, guanethidine produces an imipraminelike effect in that it enters the presynaptic sympathetic terminal by the same reuptake mechanism used to remove norepinephrine from the extracellular space. This not only explains the ability of guanethidine to potentiate the effects of exogenous norepinephrine at the same time that endogenous sympathetic function is blocked, but also may account for the initial increase in blood pressure after guanethidine. It releases endogenous norepinephrine when first given and blocks its reuptake, thereby causing an initial increase in peripheral vascular resistance. Once norepinephrine is depleted, little can be released by guanethidine or by nerve activity. Therefore, the inhibition of reuptake has no effect, and peripheral resistance and blood pressure decrease. This also illustrates why the tricyclic antidepressants, which also block norepinephrine reuptake, block guanethidine's antihypertensive effects—they block guanethidine's access to the presynaptic terminal.

Pharmacokinetics. Guanethidine is poorly absorbed after oral administration. The rate of absorption varies from 3% to 30% of the administered dose. The fact that guanethidine is a highly charged molecule explains its inability to enter the brain and its high rate of excretion by the kidney. Its pharmacologic effects outlast its presence in the plasma, probably because of sequestration in the adrenergic nerves in small but pharmacologically effective concentrations. Guanethidine is metabolized to two more polar and less active metabolites.

Adverse Effects. Since guanethidine, unlike methyldopa and clonidine, blocks sympathetic nerve function, venous pooling and orthostatic hypotension frequently occur. Ejaculatory failure also occurs, as does fluid retention if a diuretic is not given. Blockade of the norepinephrine reuptake pump by guanethidine causes an exaggerated hypertensive response to phenylephrine or other nasal decongestants, or to any other pressor amine that normally enters the sympathetic nerve terminal via the membrane reuptake mechanism.

RESERPINE

Like guanethidine, reserpine produces a slowly developing decrease in blood pressure associated with bradycardia and decreased cardiac output. It also inhibits sympathetic reflexes, thereby frequently causing orthostatic hypotension. Unlike guanethidine, however, reserpine does not produce an initial increase in blood pressure, since it does not displace norepinephrine into the synaptic cleft or block amine reuptake. It also differs from guanethidine in that it penetrates the brain, causing sedation and potentially suicidal depression.

Reserpine is used for moderate to severe hypertension, in combination with other antihypertensive drugs.

Mechanism of Action. Reserpine binds to the presynaptic storage vesicles in such a way that vesicular uptake and storage of norepinephrine is inhibited. Therefore, norepinephrine is no longer sequestered and protected from deamination by monoamine oxidase. The resulting amine depletion decreases transmitter release in response to sympathetic nerve activity. Reserpine does not prevent transmitter release (the bretyliumlike effect), nor does it block axon terminal amine reuptake (the imipraminelike effect), however. This point needs emphasis. There is vesicular uptake that involves the transport of transmitter from the intracellular (cytoplasmic) space to the intravesicular space, and there is the entirely separate process of axonal reuptake that involves the transport of transmitter from the extracellular space to the intracellular (but extravesicular) space. Reserpine inhibits vesicular uptake of amines; guanethidine and imipramine inhibit axonal reuptake of transmitter.

The actual mechanism by which reserpine inhibits granular uptake of norepinephrine probably involves the irreversible binding of reserpine to a vesicular membrane constituent. This is not a covalent interaction, however, since detergents can remove the reserpine. It seems likely that, in binding to the vesicle, reserpine may produce a conformational change in the vesicle that traps the reserpine molecule and changes the characteristics of the vesicle in such a way that it cannot take up and store amines. The decrease in norepinephrine synthesis produced by reserpine may be due in part to the inability of the vesicle to take up dopamine that is normally converted to norepinephrine within the vesicle.

Pharmacokinetics. Reserpine is absorbed from the GI tract and subjected to a first-pass effect. The elimination half-life is approximately 100 hours (range 46 to 168 hours). Reserpine crosses the placental barrier and is secreted into the milk.

Adverse Effects. Reserpine's blockade of sympathetic function may cause orthostatic hypotension, nasal congestion, impotence, GI hypersecretion, nausea, vomiting, and diarrhea. These latter GI effects are probably due to unopposed parasympathetic tone to the gut. CNS effects include drowsiness and a severe, possibly suicidal depression.

Adrenergic Receptor Antagonists

Both the β-adrenergic receptor antagonists, eg, propranolol, nadolol, and metoprolol, and the α-adrenergic receptor antagonists, eg, phentolamine, prazosin, and phenoxybenzamine, are included in this group of compounds.

PROPRANOLOL

The prototype of the β-adrenergic receptor antagonists is propranolol. It does not discriminate between β-adrenergic receptor subtypes and, therefore, interferes with all sympathetic functions that are mediated by β-adrenergic receptors, such as heart rate and contractility, glycogenolysis occurring as a result of hypoglycemia, and bronchodilatation. Thus, propranolol and other β-adrenergic receptor antagonists decrease heart rate, cardiac output, and blood pressure. These effects are minimal during rest, when there is minimal sympathetic tone to the heart. Conversely, propranolol's effects are maximal during exertion, when sympathetic drive is increased. During exercise, propranolol decreases reflex tachycardia and the cardiac response to fluid load. As a result of decreased cardiac output, sodium and water are retained; therefore, a diuretic is often used in combination with propranolol to prevent this compensatory accumulation of fluid. Since β-adrenergic receptor antagonists do not block α-adrenergic receptor–mediated responses, the compensatory response to the decreased cardiac output and blood pressure results in an increase in peripheral resistance mediated by α-adrenergic receptor activation. This causes a decrease in blood flow to all tissues except the brain.

Propranolol blocks all β-adrenergic receptors in the brain and body, and all normal physiological processes mediated by β-adrenergic receptor activation are impaired to some degree by treatment with propranolol. Epinephrine-induced lipolysis and the resulting increase in plasma fatty acids are antagonized by propranolol, as are insulin release and glycogenolysis, which increases plasma glucose concentrations. Although normal individuals do not exhibit changes in plasma insulin and glucose concentrations after the administration of propranolol, diabetics who use insulin and patients who are prone to hypoglycemia must be handled cautiously.

The other major effect of propranolol is its action on β-adrenergic receptors in the bronchi and bronchioles. β_2-Adrenergic receptors mediate catecholamine-induced bronchodilatation. Therefore, propranolol, which does not discriminate between β_1 and β_2 subtypes, increases bronchial resistance to air flow. This is apparently because there is normally sympathetic tone to this tissue. This bronchial constriction is not a problem in nonasthmatics, but it can be a potential danger to asthmatics. In these patients, the use of a more selective β_1-adrenergic receptor antagonist such as metoprolol is indicated.

Propranolol is useful in the treatment of hypertension, arrhythmias, angina, migraine, and, possibly, some psychotic disorders.

Mechanism of Action. Propranolol's molecular mechanism of action is attributed to its ability to bind competitively with β-adrenergic receptors without eliciting a biologic response. In this way, propranolol competes for β-adrenergic receptors with blood-borne epinephrine, with β-adrenergic receptor agonists (drugs), and with norepinephrine that is released from sympathetic nerve terminals. The physiological process that propranolol affects to decrease blood pressure is less clear than the molecular mechanism by which it works. Although propranolol decreases cardiac output and blood pressure, these two effects do not occur concomitantly. Since blood pressure is determined to a large extent by the tone of the vascular smooth muscle and since propranolol decreases blood pressure, it might be expected that propranolol inhibits sympathetic tone to the vasculature and causes smooth muscle relaxation, thereby decreasing resistance and lowering blood pressure. However, the sympathetic effects on vascular smooth muscle in most tissues are mediated by α-adrenergic rather than by β-adrenergic receptors. Since β-adrenergic receptor stimulation has been shown to release presynaptic norepinephrine experimentally, it has been suggested that propranolol may decrease blood pressure in part by blocking this release of norepinephrine, thereby preventing α-adrenergic receptor–mediated vasoconstriction. It has also been suggested that, because propranolol produces a greater decrease in blood pressure in patients with elevated plasma renin activity than in those with low renin activity, propranolol's antihypertensive effects may be due, in part, to suppression of the β-adrenergic receptor–mediated release of renin. The exact mechanism of propranolol's antihypertensive effects remains unclear, but a number of β-adrenergic receptor–mediated physiological processes are likely to be involved.

Propranolol's selectivity for β-adrenergic rather than α-adrenergic receptors explains why propranolol does not often cause postural hypotension. In the resting state, there is little sympathetic tone to the vascular smooth muscle. Therefore, the capacitance vessels are dilated and serve as blood storage sites when the demand for cardiac output is low. When the individual changes to the erect position, reflex sympathetic firing releases norepinephrine onto vascular α-adrenergic receptors, causing the venoconstriction necessary for increased venous return and cardiac output. Therefore, the decreased cardiac output produced by propranolol is not associated with postural hypotension.

Pharmacokinetics. Propranolol is readily absorbed after oral administration, although a large percentage of the administered dose is metabolized by the liver in its passage through the portal circulation (first-pass effect). The percentage of drug metabolized in the first pass through the liver varies greatly, which explains the large variation in plasma concentrations of drug in normal persons who receive the same dose. Propranolol is highly bound (approximately 90% to 95%) to plasma proteins. Almost completely metabolized by the liver, it is converted to a large number of compounds that are primarily eliminated by the kidney. Its half-life is 3 to 4 hours.

Adverse Effects. As mentioned earlier, propranolol's blockade of β-adrenergic receptors may lead to bronchial constriction in asthmatics, a decreased response to hypoglycemia, and heart failure in patients whose sympathetic responses are already compromised by disease or other drugs. A withdrawal syndrome can occur at the cessation of propranolol therapy; for example, individuals treated for angina or myocardial infarction can suffer severe angina or infarction upon withdrawal. Similarly, rebound hypertension can occur in patients who have taken propranolol for hypertension. Effects apparently unrelated to β-adrenergic receptor blockade include nausea, vomiting, GI upset, hallucinations, dizziness, depression, and an allergic reaction characterized by rash and fever.

NADOLOL

Like propranolol, nadolol in a nonselective, competitive, β-adrenergic receptor antagonist. It is not metabolized by the liver, however, and is excreted unchanged by the kidney. It has a long half-life (20 to 24 hours), permitting once a day dosing. Pharmacologic uses, effects, and side-effects are similar to those of propranolol.

METOPROLOL

The cardiac effects of metoprolol are the same as those of propranolol. Since metoprolol is a relatively selective β_1-adrenergic receptor antagonist, it has fewer effects on processes mediated by β_2-adrenergic receptors. Therefore, metoprolol does not prevent vasodilatation in the skeletal musculature in response to exercise, and it is less likely than propranolol to cause bronchial constriction in asthmatics. Metoprolol decreases plasma renin activity in hypertensives and inhibits the β-adrenergic receptor–mediated release of insulin in response to hypoglycemia.

Metoprolol is useful in the treatment of hypertension and is probably useful in the treatment of angina and arrhythmias.

Mechanism of Action and Pharmacokinetics. Metoprolol produces its effects by a relatively selective β_1-adrenergic receptor blockade. It must be emphasized that the selectivity between β_1- and β_2-adrenergic receptors is relative; absolute selectivity between receptor subtypes remains an as yet unattained goal.

Metoprolol is readily absorbed from the GI tract and, like propranolol, is subject to a considerable first-pass effect. The plasma half-life is approximately 3 hours, and the drug is metabolized by the liver before excretion by the kidneys.

Adverse Effects. Metoprolol has adverse effects that are similar to those of propranolol, except that there is a reduced risk of bronchoconstriction after administration of metoprolol.

PHENOXYBENZAMINE

Blood pressure is decreased by phenoxybenzamine via vasodilatation in resistance and capacitance vessels. Since phenoxybenzamine acts by blocking α-adrenergic responses, its ability to decrease blood pressure is dependent on the amount of tonic sympathetic activity to the vascular smooth muscle. Therefore, phenoxybenzamine produces little effect when the patient is at rest. When the patient is in the erect position, however, blood pooling in the capacitance vessels as a result of α-adrenergic receptor blockade commonly causes orthostatic hypotension. In addition, reflex tachycardia is a prominent feature of α-adrenergic receptor blockade, since sympathetic cardiac reflexes are intact and mediated by β-adrenergic receptors. The antihypertensive effects of phenoxybenzamine last 3 to 4 days after a single dose.

Phenoxybenzamine is used in the treatment of the hypertension associated with pheochromocytoma, an adrenal tumor that secretes catecholamines in such concentrations that excessive α-adrenergic receptor stimulation leads to increased vasoconstriction and elevated blood pressure.

Mechanism of Action. Phenoxybenzamine binds to the same site on the α-adrenergic receptor that binds norepinephrine and other agonists and antagonists. After an initially competitive binding process, a covalent bond forms between phenoxybenzamine and the α-adrenergic receptor, resulting in irreversible, noncompetitive α-adrenergic receptor blockade.

Pharmacokinetics. Phenoxybenzamine is absorbed from the GI tract, but only 20% to 30% of the administered dose is absorbed in the active form. Small amounts of the drug remain in the body for 1 week or more, presumably as a result of covalent binding.

Adverse Effects. Reflex tachycardia as a result of decreased blood pressure and decreased venous return is common after the administration of phenoxybenzamine, as is postural hypotension due to blood pooling in the capacitance vessels.

PHENTOLAMINE

A competitive α-adrenergic receptor antagonist, phentolamine produces effects similar to those produced by phenoxybenzamine. These include decreased peripheral resistance, vasodilatation of venous capacitance vessels, decreased blood pressure, reflex tachycardia, and postural hypotension.

Phentolamine can be used in the treatment of hypertensive crisis associated with pheochromocytoma, sympathomimetic overdose, and interactions associated with the use of monoamine oxidase inhibitors.

Mechanism of Action and Pharmacokinetics. Phentolamine is a competitive α-adrenergic receptor antagonist. It is readily absorbed from the GI tract, but absorption is slow and renal excretion is rapid. Parenteral injection is needed to reach effective concentrations rapidly for the treatment of hypertensive crisis. Phentolamine is secreted into the urine via the acid transport system.

Adverse Effects. Phentolamine may cause tachycardia, anginal pain, arrhythmias, GI pain, nausea, vomiting, and diarrhea.

PRAZOSIN

A recently developed antihypertensive drug, prazosin seems to act by antagonism of α-adrenergic receptors, but it does not produce marked reflex tachycardia. Prazosin decreases vascular tone in the peripheral resistance and capacitance vessels, thus decreasing venous return, cardiac output, and blood pressure. Chronic use of prazosin reduces peripheral resistance and blood pressure, but causes relatively small changes in cardiac output or heart rate. Because initial dosing with prazosin can cause postural hypotension, it is preferable to begin therapy before sleep, when the risk of postural hypotension is reduced.

Prazosin is useful in the treatment of hypertension.

Mechanism of Action. Recent evidence suggests that prazosin is a relatively specific antagonist at α_1-adrenergic receptors (postsynaptic receptors) with little affinity for α_2-adrenergic receptors (presynaptic receptors that may modulate norepinephrine release). It has been suggested that prazosin does not cause marked reflex tachycardia because of this hypothesized selectivity. According to this view, prazosin leaves presynaptic receptors unblocked. When reflex sympathetic activity occurs in response to prazosin's effects on peripheral resistance and blood pressure, the norepinephrine released from the terminal is free to interact with the presynaptic α_2-adrenergic receptors, thereby feedback-inhibiting its own release. Regardless of the reason that prazosin does not produce marked reflex tachycardia, it is an important difference between prazosin and other α-adrenergic antagonists.

Pharmacokinetics. Prazosin is absorbed from the GI tract and probably subjected to a first-pass effect. It is virtually completely metabolized by the liver, and its half-life is approximately 3 hours.

Adverse Effects. When therapy is initiated, prazosin causes drowsiness, palpitations, dizziness, fatigue, and postural hypotension. The incidence of these side-effects is usually less with prazosin than with other α-adrenergic receptor antagonists, however.

Smooth Muscle Vasodilators

HYDRALAZINE

Peripheral vascular resistance and blood pressure are decreased by hydralazine; heart rate, stroke volume, and cardiac output are increased. Hydralazine produces greater vasodilatation of the arterioles than of the capacitance vessels. Therefore, postural hypotension is minimized, since there is less blood pooling. Even though cardiac output is not decreased, reflex tachycardia occurs. Reflex sympathetic activity is apparently responsible for the increase in plasma renin activity produced by hydralazine. Sodium and water are retained, but other parameters of renal function, eg, renal tubular filtration and glomerular filtration, are not affected significantly. Interestingly, the antihypertensive effects of hydralazine take 15 to 20 minutes to occur, even after IV injection.

Hydralazine is useful in the treatment of essential hypertension. It is often used in combination with a β-adrenergic receptor antagonist, since this blocks the reflex tachycardia and the increase in plasma renin that hydralazine induces. Hydralazine can also be used for treating hypertensive emergencies, although the onset of action is slower than that of diazoxide.

Mechanism of Action. Hydralazine is a direct-acting arterial smooth muscle vasodilator, but the molecular mechanism by which hydralazine causes smooth muscle relaxation is unclear.

Pharmacokinetics. Hydralazine is absorbed from the GI tract and subjected to an extensive first-pass effect. The hepatic metabolism of hydralazine is predominantly an acetylation reaction. Patients fall into one of two genetic groups, fast acetylators and slow acetylators. Because the fast acetylators metabolize hydralazine at a more rapid rate than do slow acetylators, less of the administered dose is available to produce the desired pharmacologic effects in these patients. More importantly, those individuals who are slow acetylators experience higher hydralazine concentrations and are, therefore, more likely to suffer from a reversible lupus erythematosis–like syndrome. The plasma half-life of hydralazine is approximately 3 hours (range 2 to 8 hours). Metabolites, plus a small percentage of unchanged drug, are excreted by the kidney.

Adverse Effects. Hydralazine causes reflex tachycardia, anginal pain, anorexia, nausea, dizziness, and sweating. These effects can be prevented or decreased by combination therapy with a β-adrenergic receptor antagonist. Effects such as fever and rash, GI hemorrhage, anemia, and pancytopenia are rare; when they do occur, hydralazine therapy must be terminated. A lupuslike syndrome can also be caused by hydralazine.

DIAZOXIDE

Like hydralazine, diazoxide is a direct-acting smooth muscle vasodilator that acts preferentially on arteries and arterioles; it has little effect on venous capacitance vessels. Reflex sympathetic activity to the heart causes tachycardia and increases stroke volume and cardiac output. Since diazoxide does not dilate venous capacitance vessels, venous return is not decreased; therefore, there is little risk of postural hypotension. Sodium and water accumulate, but these compensatory effects can be prevented by concurrent use of a thiazide diuretic. Unlike hydralazine, diazoxide's antihypertensive effects are immediate. The decrease in blood pressure induced by diazoxide lasts approximately 12 hours.

Diazoxide is used to treat hypertensive emergencies and hypoglycemia.

Mechanism of Action. Diazoxide causes vasodilatation by an incompletely understood mechanism that involves a direct action on smooth muscle. It has an inhibitory effect not only on vascular smooth muscle, but also on other smooth muscle. Because of its effects on the uterus, it has been suggested that diazoxide may be useful to arrest labor.

Pharmacokinetics. After IV injection, which is the route by which diazoxide is used to treat hypertension, the volume of distribution is approximately 20% of body weight, meaning that diazoxide is not widely distributed. Diazoxide is highly protein bound (approximately 90%) and competes with orally active anticoagulants and other acidic drugs for protein binding sites. The half-life is approximately 25 hours.

Adverse Effects. Diazoxide can cause an abrupt decrease in blood pressure that can result in potentially dangerous myocardial or cerebral ischemia. Reflex sympathetic activity as a result of decreased blood pressure can cause tachycardia. Sodium and water may be retained, but such retention can be treated with a diuretic. Extravasation of the alkaline solvent in which diazoxide is dissolved can cause severe pain at the injection site.

SODIUM NITROPRUSSIDE

Unlike hydralazine and diazoxide, nitroprusside affects both arteriolar and venous smooth muscle. Therefore, nitroprusside decreases blood pressure, causes reflex tachycardia, and decreases venous return, sometimes causing postural hypotension. Not only venous return, but also cardiac work is reduced; therefore, myocardial ischemia does not occur, a fact important in the treatment of patients with impaired cardiac function. Whereas hydralazine and diazoxide can cause anginal pain, nitroprusside improves angina by decreasing cardiac return and, therefore, cardiac work. Nitroprusside's effect is immediate and outlasts an IV infusion only by minutes (its half-life is in minutes). Thus, a patient can be carefully titrated by a controlled rate of infusion, and the effect of the drug can be terminated exactly when desired.

Nitroprusside, which can be given only by IV infusion, is used to treat hypertensive emergencies, because its action is immediate. It is also used to treat acute myocardial infarction and acute congestive heart failure.

Mechanism of Action and Pharmacokinetics. Nitroprusside decreases blood pressure by a direct action on arterial and venous smooth muscle. It is very rapidly converted to thiocyanate via cyanide, which is an intermediate. Nitroprusside has a plasma half-life of a few minutes, and thiocyanate is cleared slowly by the kidney (half-life 4 hours). If kidney function is impaired, thiocyanate accumulates.

Adverse Effects. Nitroprusside's adverse effects are related to excessive vasodilatation and hypotension. They include nausea, vomiting, sweating, restlessness, headache, palpitations, and substernal distress. If thiocyanate accumulates because of renal failure, nitroprusside can cause weakness, hypoxia, tinnitus, muscle spasms, nausea, and psychosis.

Drugs That Antagonize the Renin-Angiotensin System

CAPTOPRIL

By decreasing total peripheral resistance, captopril decreases both systolic and diastolic blood pressure. It is more effective against hypertension associated with a high renin level than in hypertension due to renal failure or primary hyperaldosteronism. Captopril is effective in reducing blood pressure, however, regardless of the preexisting plasma renin activity. During treatment with captopril, plasma renin activity rises, plasma aldosterone falls, and peptidyl dipeptidase (converting enzyme) is inhibited. The plasma potassium level is elevated, and minor reflex tachycardia occurs, probably as a result of the decrease in blood pressure. Cardiac output is normal, and there is little additional retention of sodium and water.

Captopril is useful in the treatment of chronic hypertension and possibly in shock due to acute renal failure.

Mechanism of Action. Captopril inhibits peptidyl dipeptidase (converting enzyme) within minutes of administration. Because this enzyme converts angiotensin I to angiotensin II and inhibits the degradation of bradykinin, its inhibition decreases the concentration of angiotensin II and increases that of bradykinin. Captopril does not block the effects of exogenous angiotensin II, but it potentiates the effects of exogenous bradykinin. It is generally believed that captopril decreases blood pressure by inhibiting peptidyl dipeptidase. According to this view, the decrease in blood pressure is secondary to reduced angiotensin II concentrations or an increased bradykinin concentration. However, recent results show that, in the interval between doses of captopril, peptidyl dipeptidase resumes normal activity (although blood pressure remains depressed). This lack of correlation between enzyme inhibition and decreased blood pressure may be explainable in terms of a secondary process related to enzyme inhibition, or captopril's antihypertensive activity may be unrelated to its inhibition of peptidyl dipeptidase. This uncertainty about captopril's precise mechanism of action is typical of new drugs and will undoubtedly be elucidated by further research.

Pharmacokinetics. Captopril is readily absorbed from the GI tract. It is 25% to 30% bound to plasma proteins, and its plasma half-life is approximately 2 hours. Half of the administered dose is excreted by the kidneys unchanged. The remainder of the drug is in the forms of the disulphide dimer of captopril and captopril-cysteine disulfide.

Adverse Effects. Proteinuria, neutropenia, rash, pruritus, fever, hypotension, palpitations, and loss of taste perception, possibly leading to anorexia, may occur with chronic captopril therapy. The incidence of these effects is low, however.

DIURETICS

Benzothiadiazides

Chlorothiazide is the prototype drug of benzothiadiazides, which include chlorothiazide, hydrochlorothiazide, hydroflumethiazide, bendroflumethiazide, benzthiazide, methyclothiazide, polythiazide, trichlormethiazide, chlorthalidone, metolazone, quinethazone, and acetazolamide. Chlorothiazide, discussed here as representative of the group, causes an initial decrease in blood volume and cardiac output. During chronic therapy, peripheral resistance, plasma volume, and blood pressure decrease, but cardiac output returns to normal. Sodium excretion is increased, which is apparently a causative factor in the antihypertensive effects of the thiazide diuretics. Replacement of excreted water or infusion with dextran does not reverse chlorothiazide's antihypertensive effects, although sodium replacement reverses this effect. The fact that chlorothiazide's antihypertensive effect does not take place in anephric animals suggests that chlorothiazide acts primarily in the kidney to increase sodium and water excretion, which results in decreased plasma volume, peripheral vasodilatation, and decreased blood pressure.

Thiazide diuretics are used as the mainstay of antihypertensive therapy and can be effective when used alone in mild hypertensive states.

Mechanism of Action. Thiazides increase the excretion of sodium and water by a direct action on the kidney. They enter the tubular fluid by glomerular filtration and by active secretion via the acid transport system. It is apparently by this latter, competitive mechanism that thiazides block uric acid secretion, thereby elevating the plasma uric acid concentration. The precise mechanism by which thiazides block sodium reabsorption is unknown, but it appears to involve an action on the distal tubule segment that normally reabsorbs sodium and on the last 20% of the proximal tubule. Since thiazides do not abolish the renal osmotic gradient, it is inferred that they do not affect the ascending loop of Henle. Thiazides also increase the urinary excretion of potassium; this effect may be reduced during chronic therapy, however. The hypotensive effects of the thiazide diuretics are believed to result from decreased peripheral vascular resistance that, in turn, is believed to occur in response to the decreased level of sodium. Thiazides may also have a direct vasodilator action in the vascular smooth muscle.

Pharmacokinetics. Thiazides are readily absorbed from the GI tract and are variably bound by plasma proteins. Chlorothiazide distributes throughout the extracellular water and is actively accumulated only by the kidney. Most thiazides are rapidly excreted in the urine. Exceptions are bendroflumethiazide, chlorthalidone, metolazone, and polythiazide, which are excreted more slowly and, therefore, have a longer duration of action.

Adverse Effects. Hypersensitivity reactions to thiazides have been reported, as have purpura, dermatitis, and necrotizing vasculitis. Hypokalemia, hyperglycemia, and hyperuricemia can occur. Hypokalemia is observed to some degree in most patients, but it is negligible when the patients are given an adequate diet, including fruit. Reduction of thiazide dose is preferable to routine potassium supplementation.

Loop Diuretics

Furosemide and ethacrynic acid, called loop diuretics or high-ceiling diuretics, differ from the thiazides in that they produce a more marked diuresis more quickly (within 30 minutes) than do the thiazides. Sodium, potassium, magnesium, calcium, and water excretion is greatly increased. Since these acids are secreted into the tubular lumen via the acid transport mechanism, secretion of uric acid is inhibited competitively, leading to hyperuricemia. Phosphate excretion is often decreased.

Loop diuretics are useful in the treatment of edema, whether it is of renal, hepatic, or cardiac origin. Furosemide and ethacrynic acid are useful in treating acute pulmonary edema when the amount of body fluid must be reduced immediately and in severe anemia when the increased blood volume resulting from transfusion might cause cardiac failure. These compounds can also be used to treat hypertension in patients with impaired renal function.

Mechanism of Action. Loop diuretics block sodium reabsorption in the ascending loop of Henle, thereby abolishing the osmotic gradient in the kidney. The efficacy of furosemide and ethacrynic acid is, therefore, greater than that of the thiazides, which do not abolish the osmotic gradient. Loop diuretics have been shown to act on the proximal and distal tubules, but the main effect of these diuretics is believed to be blockade of sodium transport into the cells of the ascending limb. The molecular mechanism of action is unclear but may involve inhibition of chloride transport (thereby blocking NaCl absorption) and an inhibitory action on kidney Na^+-K^+-dependent ATPase.

Pharmacokinetics. Furosemide is given by both oral and parenteral routes. It is readily absorbed from the GI tract and bound by plasma proteins. Furosemide is excreted into the urine by glomerular filtration and via the acid secretion mechanism. A small fraction of administered drug is metabolized by cleavage of the side chain, and some is excreted in the feces.

Ethacrynic acid is also absorbed readily from the GI tract and highly bound to plasma proteins. After IV injection, ethacrynic acid is metabolized by the liver (approximately one third), and the remainder is excreted by the kidney.

Adverse Effects. Furosemide is more commonly used than ethacrynic acid, because the incidence of GI side-effects is lower with furosemide. The main adverse effect of these highly efficacious diuretics, ie, electrolyte imbalance, is related to their mechanism of action. In addition, irreversible deafness is an uncommon but major complication. Furosemide is known to cause fetal and maternal death in animals.

Aldosterone Antagonists: Spironolactone

The antihypertensive properties of spironolactone are similar to those of the thiazide diuretics. Spironolactone increases sodium and water excretion and decreases blood pressure. Spironolactone and the thiazides differ primarily in their effects on potassium excretion. Whereas thiazides increase potassium excretion, spironolactone is less likely to cause hypokalemia and can even cause hyperkalemia. Since spironolactone commonly produces undesirable side-effects at antihypertensive doses, it should be used only when thiazides are contraindicated.

Spironolactone is useful in the treatment of hypertension, refractory edema, and other disorders in which blockade of aldosterone-mediated responses is desired.

Mechanism of Action. Spironolactone is a competitive aldosterone receptor antagonist. Aldosterone normally increases sodium and water uptake by the distal tubule, as well as the excretion of potassium by cells of the distal nephron. Stimuli to aldosterone release include decreased blood volume, hyponatremia, hyperkalemia, and angiotensin II receptor activation. Therefore, aldosterone receptor antagonism by spironolactone blocks sodium and water absorption, as well as potassium excretion by the kidney.

Pharmacokinetics. Spironolactone is readily absorbed from the GI tract, and its bioavailability is about 90%. The drug is more than 90% bound to plasma proteins, and it is rapidly and extensively metabolized, primarily to the active metabolite canrenone, which has a plasma half-life of 12 to 24 hours. It is excreted in the urine and bile.

Adverse Effects. Spironolactone commonly causes gynecomastia. It also produces hyperkalemia and GI symptoms. A carcinogenic action of spironolactone is likely. The frequency of side-effects when spironolactone is used and the availability of other equally efficacious and less toxic drugs suggest that spironolactone should be used only when alternatives are unacceptable in specific cases.

Potassium-Sparing Diuretics

TRIAMTERENE

Triamterene increases the excretion of sodium, chloride, and water and slightly alkalinizes the urine. Potassium excretion is slightly increased when triamterene is given alone; in combination therapy with another saluretic, however, potassium excretion is often decreased markedly, which can lead to hyperkalemia.

Triamterene is useful in the treatment of edema, but not in the treatment of hypertension. It is often used in combination with other diuretics to produce an additive diuretic effect and to decrease potassium loss.

Mechanism of Action. Triamterene blocks the absorption of sodium and chloride by an action on the kidney. Potassium secretion by the distal nephron is decreased. The molecular mechanism by which triamterene blocks sodium and chloride absorption is unclear, but it does not appear to involve aldosterone receptor antagonism.

Pharmacokinetics. Triamterene is absorbed from the GI tract, and approximately half is bound to plasma proteins. Triamterene and active metabolites are excreted in the urine after glomerular filtration and tubular secretion.

Adverse Effects. The major adverse effect of triamterene is hyperkalemia. Other effects include nausea, vomiting, dizziness, leg cramps, and reversible azotemia, although these are uncommon.

AMILORIDE

Like spironolactone and triamterene, amiloride is a potassium-sparing diuretic. It increases sodium, chloride, and water excretion, but decreases potassium secretion. Slight alkalinization of the urine occurs, probably as a result of decreased hydrogen ion secretion.

Amiloride is useful in the treatment of edema, often in combination with a thiazide. Its mechanism of action is the same as that of triamterene.

Amiloride is absorbed from the GI tract. It produces peak diuresis 6 to 10 hours after administration and its effects last for 24 hours. Plasma half-life is 6 to 9 hours. Amiloride is excreted unchanged by the kidney.

5

Drugs That Affect Uterine Motility

Since the motility of uterine smooth muscle must be kept under strong physiological control during pregnancy and labor, it is the target of many inputs, both neural and humoral. Therefore, uterine smooth muscle cells possess many receptors for endogenous ligands that increase or decrease uterine motility. The uterus receives parasympathetic innervation, which produces variable effects, as well as sympathetic innervation. Activation of α-adrenergic receptors stimulates uterine activity; activation of β-adrenergic receptors inhibits uterine activity. In addition to cholinergic and adrenergic receptors, uterine muscle contains receptors for steroid hormones, oxytocin, prostaglandins, serotonin, histamine, and, no doubt, many other endogenous molecules.

ERGOT ALKALOIDS

The pharmacologic and toxicologic effects of the ergot alkaloids have been known and utilized for more than 2,500 years. Ergots comprise a group of compounds produced by the fungus *Claviceps purpurea,* which grows primarily on rye grain in wet conditions. Ergot poisoning causes vomiting, diarrhea, unquenchable thirst, formication (the feeling that bugs are crawling on the skin), itching, cold and numb skin and limbs, muscle pain, abortion, confusion, drowsiness, and convulsions. Chronic decreases in blood flow to the arms and legs lead, in severe cases, to limb death and detachment without loss of blood. The blackening and drying of the limbs have been compared to the effects of fire in producing charcoal; ergotism was therefore called St. Anthony's Fire in the Middle Ages, since a visit to St. Anthony's shrine was said to be curative. In addition to divine intervention, the ergot-free diet that was eaten while visiting the shrine may have contributed to the relief of symptoms.

Recently, a retrospective study of the Salem witch trials of the 17th century suggested that the bewitching symptoms suffered by a number of people (sickness of the stomach, lameness, pain in the legs and feet, pinching and prickling sensation, and convulsions) may have been due to ergotism rather than bedevilment. The year of the witchcraft trials (1691–1692) coincided with a cold winter followed by a wet spring, conditions that favor fungal growth on rye grain, a crop known to have been grown in the area.

The medical use of ergots to induce labor began in the early 19th century, but they were almost certainly used illicitly as an abortifacient long before then. Subsequent chemical identification and synthesis showed that ergot consisted of the ergot alkaloids (congeners of d-lysergic acid) and simpler amines, eg, histamine, tyramine, and choline. The ergot alkaloids used clinically include ergotamine, dihydroergotamine, and methysergide, which are used in treating migraine headaches; bromocriptine, which is used in treating galactorrhea and possibly parkinsonism; and ergonovine and methylergonovine, which are used in obstetric practice.

While uterine sensitivity to oxytocin develops only as pregnancy nears fullterm, the uterus is sensitive to ergots before, during, and after pregnancy. Sensitivity to ergots increases as gestation progresses. Shortly after oral or parenteral administration of ergonovine or methylergonovine, which have similar effects on uterine activity, uterine contractions follow intervals of relaxation; the baseline uterine tone is increased. Higher doses cause a sustained contraction. This uterotonic effect shortens the third stage of labor and decreases postpartum bleeding. Since ergots cause a sustained contraction, they are used only after delivery of the fetus. Uterotonic doses do not usually cause marked cardiovascular effects, but higher doses cause severe peripheral vasoconstriction and, therefore, increased blood pressure.

Ergonovine and methylergonovine are useful in treating postpartum hemorrhage and uterine atony.

MECHANISM OF ACTION

Ergot alkaloids are believed to produce their uterotonic and cardiovascular effects directly, primarily via an α-adrenergic receptor agonist action, since the α-adrenergic receptor antagonist phentolamine blocks the ergot's uterotonic effects. Ergots also have mixed agonist and antagonist effects on serotonin receptors, but their role in uterine contraction is unclear.

PHARMACOKINETICS

Ergonovine and methylergonovine are readily absorbed after oral administration. A uterotonic effect is evident within 10 minutes after oral administration. The principal route of metabolism involves ring hydroxylation and excretion in the bile. The duration of action is several hours.

ADVERSE EFFECTS

Ergotism due to chronic ingestion is not likely to occur when ergots are used acutely to increase uterine activity. However, ergots can cause vomiting and a 20 mm Hg rise in blood pressure.

OXYTOCIN

An endogenous eight amino acid–containing peptide hormone, oxytocin is synthesized in the paraventricular and supraoptic nuclei of the hypothalamus and is then transported to and released into the blood by the posterior pituitary.

The physiological role of oxytocin in labor and milk let-down has not been fully elucidated. Although exogenous oxytocin produces uterine contractions virtually indistinguishable from those observed in spontaneous labor, oxytocin concentrations in maternal plasma do not increase at the onset of labor. Some evidence suggests that oxytocin of fetal, rather than maternal, origin may play a causative role in the induction of labor. Unlike the ergots, oxytocin does not stimulate uterine activity at all times during gestation. Before and during the early part of pregnancy, the uterus is relatively insensitive to oxytocin. Sensitivity develops progressively throughout pregnancy, particularly in the third trimester, apparently because of an increase in the density of uterine oxytocin receptors.

Oxytocin not only increases the frequency and force of uterine contraction, but also stimulates the myoepithelial tissue of the alveoli in the breast. This contraction moves the milk from the alveoli to the large ducts for subsequent suckling. Oxytocin has weak but significant effects on vascular smooth muscle and on the kidney. In high doses, oxytocin can cause peripheral vasodilatation, increased blood flow, and decreased blood pressure. Oxytocin has weak vasopressinlike activity, causing an antidiuretic effect in large doses.

Oxytocin is used to induce labor, to decrease postpartum hemorrhage, for uterine atony, and to stimulate milk let-down.

MECHANISM OF ACTION

The myometrial cells of the uterus contain oxytocin receptors on their outer surfaces. Stimulation of these receptors by oxytocin causes depolarization, increased spike production, and increased smooth muscle contraction. This process involves sodium and calcium influx and may involve a prostaglandin mediator. The gradually increasing uterine sensitivity to oxytocin during gestation is paralleled by an increase in the number of oxytocin receptors in the uterus. Estrogen, which is known to potentiate oxytocin's uterotonic effect, may play a role in this increasing sensitivity. Milk let-down is produced by a similar oxytocin receptor–mediated mechanism, and the antidiuretic effect is due to weak antidiuretic hormone agonist actions in the kidney.

PHARMACOKINETICS

Oxytocin is administered by parenteral (including nasal) routes. It has a half-life between less than a minute to several minutes. It is metabolized by the liver, kidney, and mammary gland, as well as by plasma oxytocinase.

ADVERSE EFFECTS

The main adverse effects of oxytocin are related to its uterotonic action. These can include uterine rupture, fetal death, and pelvic hematoma. Also reported are nausea, vomiting, premature ventricular contractions, anaphylactic reactions, hypertensive episodes, and water intoxication.

PROSTAGLANDINS

It is now believed that prostaglandins play an important role in the labor process. Endogenous prostaglandin E_2 (PGE$_2$) and prostaglandin $F_{2\alpha}$ (PGF$_{2\alpha}$) are present in the uterus and amniotic fluid, and their concentration in umbilical blood and amniotic fluid is elevated at labor. Exogenous PGE$_2$ and PGF$_{2\alpha}$ increase uterine contraction. Aspirinlike drugs, which decrease prostaglandin synthesis, delay and prolong labor. The uterus is sensitive to the uterotonic effects of PGE$_2$ and PGF$_{2\alpha}$ before, during, and after pregnancy. It has been suggested that endogenous prostaglandins may mediate oxytocin's uterotonic effects, because oxytocin releases prostaglandins and because inhibition of prostaglandin synthesis decreases oxytocin's contractile effects in vivo and in vitro. In addition, recent evidence suggests that a factor present in fetal urine (possibly a small lipid or steroid) may trigger the onset of labor by stimulating prostaglandin synthesis in the fetal membranes.

Prostaglandin E_2 and $F_{2\alpha}$ are used clinically to stimulate uterine activity. They are effective for inducing labor or abortion. The uterotonic effects of the prostaglandins are qualitatively similar to those of oxytocin, but the effects of the prostaglandins last longer. The main difference between the effects of prostaglandins and those of oxytocin is that, during the early stages of pregnancy, the uterus responds to prostaglandins while responses to oxytocin are virtually absent. Prostaglandins produce uterine contraction that can lead to uterine hypertonus and abnormal contraction complexes.

MECHANISM OF ACTION

The exact molecular mechanism by which prostaglandins produce uterine contraction is unknown. Since prostaglandins are synthesized, released, and degraded locally, exogenous prostaglandins presumably act directly on the tissue where the endogenous prostaglandins act to cause uterine contractions. It is presently believed that prostaglandins act on membrane-associated receptors that are specific for endogenous prostaglandins. Prostaglandins apparently increase sodium and calcium influx, thus causing an increase in excitation-contraction coupling. Electrophysiological studies show that prostaglandins depolarize uterine cells and increase spike frequency.

PHARMACOKINETICS

Prostaglandins are absorbed after any route of administration. Since intramuscular and subcutaneous injection of prostaglandins is extremely painful, prostaglandins are given orally, intravenously, or locally (into the vagina, uterus, or amniotic fluid). Prostaglandins given systemically are metabolized rapidly, particularly by the lung.

ADVERSE EFFECTS

Prostaglandins can cause uterine hypertonus by their direct action on the uterus, as well as nausea, vomiting, and diarrhea by their action on intestinal smooth muscle. Tachycardia, headache, fever, and EEG changes have been reported, all presumably due to the effects of administered prostaglandins on functions normally influenced by endogenous prostaglandins.

TOCOLYTICS

Four groups of drugs inhibit uterine motility and may be useful in treating premature labor: the sympathomimetic amines, which act by stimulating uterine β-adrenergic receptors; progestins; ethanol; and inhibitors of prostaglandin synthesis.

β-Adrenergic Receptor Agonists

Uterine activity may be inhibited by a β-adrenergic receptor agonist action on postsynaptic receptors of the sympathetic input to the uterus. Histofluorescent studies show that sympathetic nerves innervate the blood vessels and smooth muscle of the uterus. Both α-adrenergic and β-adrenergic receptors are present in the uterus. Stimulation of β-adrenergic receptors by endogenously released norepinephrine and epinephrine, or by β-adrenergic receptor agonists, causes uterine muscle relaxation. This is the functional basis for the use of β-adrenergic agonists in treating premature uterine activity. In addition to their use in premature labor, β-adrenergic receptor agonists can be used to counteract the effects of excessive oxytocin infusion and to relax the uterus prior to cesarean delivery, fetoscopy, and the transport of women in labor.

RITODRINE

Like terbutaline, isoxsuprine, and other β-adrenergic receptor agonists, ritodrine inhibits uterine motility. It is a β_2-adrenergic receptor agonist. Since the β-adrenergic receptors of the uterus are of the β_2 subtype, relatively selective β_2-adrenergic receptor agonists may produce fewer cardiac side-effects mediated by the β_1 subtype. In practice, ritodrine does produce cardiac effects, such as tachycardia, although it probably produces fewer cardiac effects than does isoxsuprine. Ritodrine may inhibit uterine activity in part by decreasing concentrations of $PGF_{2\alpha}$, which may play a role in initiating or maintaining premature labor.

OTHER SYMPATHOMIMETICS

Virtually any β-adrenergic receptor agonist inhibits uterine activity, including terbutaline, albuterol, isoxsuprine, and cinnamedrine. The mechanism of action of these drugs is the same as that of ritodrine, ie, β-adrenergic receptor stimulation. Adverse cardiovascular effects as a result of β-adrenergic receptor stimulation are the major drawback to their use.

Progesterone

Because progesterone appears to play a physiological role in maintaining pregnancy, partly by inhibiting uterine contractility, it has been used to treat premature labor. The molecular mechanism by which progesterone inhibits uterine motility is unclear. It is generally believed that progesterone, like other steroids, produces its biologic effects first by entering the cell (steroids are highly lipid-soluble) and then binding with cytoplasmic steroid receptors; the steroid-receptor complex is then translocated to the nucleus. Within the nucleus, the steroid-receptor complex binds to DNA and alters RNA transcription and protein synthesis. The inhibitory effect of progesterone on uterine motility is the result of as yet unknown cellular changes. Direct effects of progesterone on membrane function and calcium influx have also been suggested. Fetal anomalies produced by exogenous progestins militate against their routine use as tocolytics.

Ethanol

Ethyl alcohol has been used to decrease uterine activity in premature labor. Intravenous infusion for hours is used to maintain plasma ethanol at 0.09% to 0.16%, an inebriating range. The mechanism by which ethanol decreases uterine motility may involve inhibition of oxytocin release by a central action of ethanol. The exact molecular mechanism by which any of ethanol's effects are produced remains obscure.

Inhibitors of Prostaglandin Synthesis

Endogenous prostaglandins are believed to play an important role in either inducing or maintaining labor; therefore, inhibitors of prostaglandin synthesis have been used to decrease uterine activity in premature labor. Indomethacin has been used with some success for treatment of premature labor.

6

Antimicrobial Agents

SULFONAMIDES

The first class of drugs to be systematically and successfully used as antibacterial agents were the sulfonamides. All sulfonamides inhibit bacterial growth (sulfonamides are only bacteriostatic) by competitive antagonism of the bacterial enzyme dihydropteroate synthetase, the enzyme that binds *p*-amino-benzoic acid (PABA) and synthesizes folic acid. All mammalian cells need folic acid for a variety of reactions, including DNA and RNA synthesis. Because mammalian cells cannot synthesize folic acid, they use folic acid obtained in the diet. Only those bacteria that require folate but cannot absorb it from the environment in which they grow must synthesize folate from PABA; therefore, only these organisms are susceptible to the bacteriostatic effects of the sulfonamides. Since the inhibition of PABA binding to dihydropteroate synthetase by sulfonamides is competitive, addition of excess PABA in vitro reverses the inhibition.

One compound often used clinically in combination with a sulfonamide is trimethoprim. Although not a sulfonamide, trimethoprim also inhibits folate synthesis. Two inhibitors of folate synthesis are used on the premise that sequential blockade of two different steps in the synthesis of folates might be advantageous clinically—it is. Trimethoprim inhibits the enzyme dihydrofolate reductase, another enzyme involved in folate metabolism. Although mammalian cells also have this enzyme, the bacterial enzyme is far more sensitive to trimethoprim than is the mammalian enzyme. Given alone, trimethoprim is weakly bacteriostatic. Given in combination with a sulfonamide, usually sulfamethoxazole, a synergistic effect is obtained.

The sulfonamides, as a class, are well absorbed orally (70% to 100% of an administered dose). The exceptions are the sulfonamides used specifically to sterilize the intestinal lumen when systemic absorption is not desired. Unlike many antibiotics, the sulfonamides distribute widely. Sulfadiazine distributes throughout the total body water, while sulfisoxazole is restricted to the extracellular water. Both drugs penetrate the brain and reach concentrations in the CSF that are effective against meningococcal infection. Equilibrium between maternal and fetal circulations takes approximately 3 hours after an oral dose, and the fetal concentration reached can be toxic.

The main route of metabolism of sulfonamides is N-acetylation by the liver, which decreases the antibacterial efficacy but not the toxicity of the molecule. The parent drug and its metabolites are excreted in the urine by glomerular filtration. Because the acetylated derivatives are often less water-soluble than the parent molecules, the derivatives are more likely to cause crystalluria and the development of crystalline aggregates throughout the urinary system. The use of more water-soluble sulfonamides, such as sulfisoxazole, largely avoids this problem. Sulfonamides can also cause acute hemolytic anemias, aplastic anemia, thrombocytopenia, eosinophilia, agranulocytosis, hypersensitivity reactions, hepatitis, nausea, vomiting, and other adverse effects.

Uses

Many of the bacteria that were once susceptible to the sulfonamides have developed into resistant forms. This may be due to the presence of an altered enzyme or to the development of the ability by some bacteria to synthesize sufficient PABA, even in the presence of a sulfonamide, for adequate folic acid synthesis. The development of resistant forms and the development of more effective, less toxic antibacterial compounds have limited the uses of the sulfonamides. Sulfonamides are presently used to treat

1. Urinary tract infections. Most urinary tract infections involve *Escherichia coli* that are still susceptible to sulfonamides. A combination of sulfamethoxazole and trimethoprim is used widely.
2. Meningococcal infection. Sulfisoxazole or sulfadiazine can be used to treat meningococcal infection when it is caused by a sulfonamide-sensitive organism or when the patient is allergic to penicillin. Sulfonamides are also useful for prophylactic treatment of individuals who expect to come in close contact with meningococci.
3. Nocardiosis. Nocardial infections can be effectively treated with sulfisoxazole or sulfadiazine.
4. Rheumatic fever prophylaxis. Sulfisoxazole is effective in the prophylactic treatment of rheumatic fever and is used primarily in patients allergic to penicillin.
5. Toxoplasmosis. Sulfadiazine is used in combination with pyrimethamine to treat toxoplasmosis.
6. Other infections. Sulfonamides are effective in treating a large variety of

other infectious disorders, but newer, more effective, and less toxic antibiotics are preferred.

Specific Compounds

Sulfisoxazole is rapidly absorbed and distributed throughout the extracellular water. The high water solubility of both the parent drug and the acetylated metabolite greatly decreases the possibility of renal crystallization, crystalluria, or anuria. Drug concentrations in urine exceed those in blood, making sulfisoxazole particularly useful for treating urinary tract infection. Sulfisoxazole is a short-acting sulfonamide (mostly excreted in 24 hours).

The main difference between sulfamethoxazole and sulfisoxazole is that the former is more slowly excreted in the urine and is, therefore, longer acting. Sulfamethoxazole is also more likely to cause crystalluria due to precipitation of the parent drug and the lower water solubility of the acetylated metabolite.

Unlike the preceding sulfonamides, sulfadiazine is distributed throughout the total body water. It is absorbed rapidly and excreted rapidly. High fluid intake and alkalinization of the urine inhibit crystalluria.

Less frequently used sulfonamides include sulfacytine and sulfamethizole (used for urinary tract infections), phthalylsulfathiazole and sulfasalazine (used to decrease bowel flora), sulfacetamide (used topically for ophthalmic infections), and silver sulfadiazine and mafenide acetate (used topically for burns).

PENICILLIN AND RELATED COMPOUNDS

The discovery of penicillin was a major breakthrough in antibiotic therapy, and penicillin remains today the drug of choice for a variety of bacterial diseases. Penicillin, its congeners, and the cephalosporins act by inhibiting the normal synthesis of the bacterial cell wall. Since the cytoplasm of penicillin-treated bacteria is hypertonic, compared with the mammalian extracellular fluid in which it grows, the cell wall no longer protects the bacterium from the effects of the osmotic gradient. Water enters down its osmotic gradient, and the cell swells and lyses. Therefore, penicillin is bacteriocidal. If, however, the bacterium is in an isotonic medium, there is no net movement of water into the bacterium, and the cell survives. In this case, penicillin is bacteriostatic.

Bacteria have a rigid cell wall that covers the cellular plasma membrane and protects them from the osmotic difference between their internal environment and the fluid in which they live. Outside the cell wall, the bacteria secrete a colloid layer, containing the proteins and other macromolecules that confer their immunologic characteristics. The cell wall is synthesized in three main steps, each of which takes place in a different location of the bacterium:

1. The first step takes place in the bacterial cytoplasm. UDP-N-acetylglucosamine is combined with a three-carbon chain and five amino acids to form UDP-acetylmuramylpentapeptide. The last pair of the five amino acids added to UDP-N-acetylglucosamine is D-alanyl-D-alanine. The antibiotic D-cycloserine, an analog of D-alanine, acts as a competitive antagonist of D-alamine on the enzymes that join the two alanine molecules together. The UDP-acetylmuramylpentapeptide is then joined via a phospholipid carrier to the plasma membrane.

2. A second sugar is added to UDP-acetylmuramylpentapeptide, and a five-glycine chain is attached to form the glycine branch that eventually cross-links to build the cell wall. The polymer formed by UDP-acetylmuramylpentapeptide, an additional sugar, and the five-glycine chain is then cleaved from the membrane-bound phospholipid carrier after translocation to the site of cell wall synthesis. This cleavage reaction is inhibited by the antibiotic vancomycin.

3. The third step takes place outside the cell wall. Each molecule of the preceding product has a five-glycine branch, plus two terminal alanine residues. The terminal glycine residue of one of these large molecules (the UDP-acetylmuramylpentapeptide-pentaglycine chain) joins with the penultimate alanine molecule when the terminal alanine residue is released. This transpeptidase reaction is inhibited by the penicillins and cephalosporins. It is believed that penicillin may acylate the active portion of the transpeptidase molecule that normally binds the D-alanyl-D-alanine residues for the pentapeptide chain.

When a penicillin-sensitive species is cultured and treated with penicillin, some of the bacteria survive. When the surviving bacteria are subsequently cultured, they are often found to be penicillin-resistant, probably because the bacteria have developed an ability to destroy penicillin, ie, they have developed a penicillinase. In other cases, however, the unkilled bacteria remain penicillin-sensitive. It appears that, for the bacterial cell wall to grow, gaps must first be made in the cell wall to permit the insertion of new wall constituents. This function is performed by mucopeptide hydrolase, an enzyme also inhibited by penicillin. When penicillin is added to a growing culture, some of the bacteria will have just completed synthesis of their cell walls and will, therefore, be unaffected by penicillin. These bacteria do not begin the cell wall synthesis process again, since their mucopeptide hydrolase is inhibited by the penicillin. When the penicillin is no longer present, these bacteria begin to grow again and therefore survive the antibiotic treatment without having become a "resistant" form. These surviving bacteria probably play a major role in reinfection.

Some species of bacteria are resistant to penicillin. One reason for species-specific susceptibility is the structure of the cell wall. Gram-negative bacteria have relatively complex outer coats that block the entry of many penicillins. Conversely, gram-positive bacteria have simpler coats that allow penicillin to reach the site of cell wall biosynthesis. The other major reason that some bacteria are insensitive to penicillin is the ability of these organisms to synthesize penicillinase or β-lactamase, enzymes that hydrolyze penicillin and thereby inactivate it.

Penicillin is widely and incorrectly thought to have negligible effects on mammalian cells. In fact, however, penicillin is a potent and highly efficacious convulsant. It produces epileptiform neuronal activity by antagonizing the protective inhibitory postsynaptic potentials generated in most neurons by inhibitory interneurons. Fortunately, penicillin does not normally enter the brain and, therefore, does not cause convulsions in normal patients. However, in any condition that impairs the blood-brain barrier, such as some types of meningitis, convulsions are an expected adverse effect of penicillin therapy.

Penicillin G and Penicillin V

Although benzylpenicillin (penicillin G) and phenoxymethylpenicillin (penicillin V) have nearly identical antibacterial spectrums, there are differences in the way they are handled by the body. Penicillin G is unstable in acid and is, therefore, destroyed to a large extent in the stomach. In contrast, penicillin V is stable in acid and, therefore, can be administered orally. Once absorbed, the two penicillins are handled in similar ways by the body. Penicillin G is the group prototype.

ORAL ABSORPTION

Penicillin G is destroyed by stomach acid. Approximately one quarter of an orally administered dose is absorbed, and peak plasma concentrations are reached 30 to 60 minutes after ingestion. Absorption is mainly from the duodenum. Penicillin G is more readily absorbed from the gut of the very young and old, since stomach acidity is decreased in these groups.

DISTRIBUTION

Penicillin G is reversibly bound to plasma albumin (approximately 65% bound, 35% free) and distributed widely. Although present in most tissues, penicillin does not enter the brain and is found only in low concentration in the CSF.

EXCRETION

The main route of penicillin excretion is the kidney. Penicillin enters the urine by glomerular filtration and active acid secretion. The rapid excretion of penicillin and the resulting short duration of its action made it necessary to develop methods to prolong its stay in the plasma. In addition to the use of depot forms, the secretion of penicillin into the urine can be antagonized by the administration of probenecid, a drug that competes for the renal acid transport mechanism and thereby raises the concentration of penicillin in the plasma. Since 90% of excreted penicillin enters the urine by tubular secretion, this is an effective way of prolonging penicillin's stay in the body. Obviously, renal impairment also prolongs penicillin's duration of action.

ANTIBACTERIAL SPECTRUM

Penicillins G and V are still the drugs of choice for a wide variety of bacterial infections. Sensitive strains include the gram-positive bacteria *Staphylococcus aureus, Streptococcus pyogenes, Streptococcus bovis, Streptococcus pneumoniae, Streptococcus* (viridans group), *Bacillus anthracis, Clostridium perfringens, Clostridium tetani, Listeria monoctyogenes*, and *Corynebacterium diphtheriae*. Penicillin is also the drug of choice for treating infection with the gram-negative bacteria *Neisseria gonorrhoeae, Neisseria meningitidis, Fusobacterium, Leptotrichia buccalis, Pasteurella multocida, Streptobacillus moniliformis*, and *Spirillum minus*. Infections with the *Treponema* spirochetes and *Actinomyces israelii* are also treated effectively with penicillin.

Penicillinase-Resistant Penicillins

Methicillin, oxacillin, cloxacillin, dicloxacillin, floxacillin, and nafcillin are penicillinase-resistant penicillins. Although they are not as active as penicillin G against bacteria that are penicillin-sensitive, they are effective in treating bacteria that produce a penicillinase, particularly the resistant staphylococci.

METHICILLIN

The only penicillinase-resistant penicillin that is not used orally is methicillin; it is susceptible to stomach acid. Because methicillin is excreted rapidly by the kidney, parenteral injection is frequently necessary. Methicillin is ineffective against gram-negative bacteria. It is distributed and excreted as penicillin G is.

OXACILLIN, CLOXACILLIN, DICLOXACILLIN, AND FLOXACILLIN

The four penicillin congeners oxacillin, cloxacillin, dicloxacillin, and floxacillin are stable in acid and are therefore effective when administered orally. They are primarily useful in the treatment of infections due to penicillin-resistant *Staphylococcus* and are not effective against gram-negative bacteria. These drugs are rapidly excreted by the kidney (plasma half-lives are 30 to 60 minutes), so concomitant treatment with probenecid prolongs their duration of action. Unlike penicillin, these drugs are eliminated to a significant degree by hepatic secretion into the bile.

NAFCILLIN

Despite its classification as an oral penicillin congener, nafcillin is erratically absorbed from the gut. It is actively sequestered in the liver and is highly protein bound. It is largely excreted by the liver; only 10% of an administered dose appears in the urine, and concomitant administration of probenecid further decreases this proportion. Nafcillin, unlike other penicillins, reaches therapeutic concentrations in the CSF. It is more effective against penicillinase-producing *Staphylococcus* than the other drugs of the class.

Broad Spectrum Penicillins

Addition of a single amino group to the penicillin G molecule yields ampicillin, prototype of a class of antibiotics with considerable efficacy against gram-negative bacteria. Congeners of ampicillin include amoxicillin, hetacillin, pivampicillin, carbenicillin, mezlocillin, piperacillin, and ticarcillin. Like penicillin itself, all these derivatives of penicillin are susceptible to penicillinase and are, therefore, of little value against staphylococcal infections. Although effective against the gram-positive bacteria that are penicillin-sensitive, ampicillin is less potent than penicillin G against these organisms. Ampicillin and its congeners are particularly effective in treating infection with enterococci, *Listeria monocytogenes, Proteus mirabilis, Haemophilus influenzae,* and *Salmonella.* The number of resistant strains has increased with increased use of these compounds, however. Most of the congeners of ampicillin have an antibacterial spectrum similar to that of ampicillin, although carbenicillin, ticarcillin, mezlocillin, and piperacillin are effective against *Pseudomonas, Klebsiella,* and some other ampicillin-resistant strains.

AMPICILLIN

As it is stable in acid, ampicillin is readily absorbed from the gastrointestinal (GI) tract. Like penicillin, ampicillin is rapidly excreted in the urine via tubular secretion. Concomitant treatment with penicillin or probenecid prolongs ampicillin's duration of action by competition for the acid secretory process in the kidney. Ampicillin is also metabolized by the liver, but renal dysfunction greatly increases its half-life in the body.

AMOXICILLIN

Addition of a hydroxyl group to ampicillin yields amoxicillin, a penicillinase-sensitive drug that has pharmacologic and pharmacokinetic properties similar to those of ampicillin. Amoxicillin is less effective than ampicillin against *Shigella* and somewhat more effective against enterococci and *Salmonella.* It is also more readily absorbed than ampicillin after oral administration.

HETACILLIN AND PIVAMPICILLIN

Both hetacillin and pivampicillin are converted to ampicillin in vivo and, therefore, have little advantage over ampicillin.

CARBENICILLIN

The main advantage of carbenicillin is its efficacy (in high doses) against *Pseudomonas.* Because it is both acid-sensitive and penicillinase-sensitive, it is used only by the parenteral route. It is excreted by the kidney, but its presence can be prolonged by concomitant treatment with probenecid. Carbenicillin inactivates aminoglycosides if the two solutions are mixed together.

TICARCILLIN, MEZLOCILLIN, AND PIPERACILLIN

The newer antibiotics, ie, ticarcillin, mezlocillin, and piperacillin, are similar to carbenicillin; however, they are much more potent than carbenicillin against *Pseudomonas.* Ticarcillin is four times more potent against *Pseudomonas* than carbenicillin, and mezlocillin is ten times more potent than carbenicillin. Mezlocillin is also effective against *Klebsiella.* Piperacillin is the most potent agent in the class against many varieties of *Enterobacteriaceae,* including *Klebsiella.* All three are sensitive to penicillinase and are handled by the body as penicillin is handled.

Cephalosporins

The antibiotics known as cephalosporins are derived from cephalosporin C, one of three antibiotics produced by the fungus *Cephalosporium acremonium.* Cephalosporins block bacterial cell wall synthesis and appear to have the same mechanism of action as penicillin. Also like the penicillins, cephalosporins are excreted by the kidney via glomerular filtration and active tubular secretion that is blocked competitively by probenecid. Unlike penicillin, however, the cephalosporins are active against both gram-negative and gram-positive bacteria; in addition, they are resistant to penicillinase. Some cephalosporins are susceptible to β-lactamase–producing bacteria, eg, *Klebsiella airogenes* and *Pseudomonas aeruginosa.* Cephalosporins do not enter cells, nor do they enter the brain. Cephalosporins reach therapeutically effective concentrations in lung, muscle, kidney, bone, placenta, synovial fluid, and pericardial fluid. Low concentrations are present in the humors of the eye.

ABSORPTION

Cephalexin, cephradine, cefaclor, and cefadroxil are readily absorbed from the gut and can therefore be used orally. Cephalothin and cephapirin are given only by the intravenous route, since intramuscular injection is painful and they are not readily absorbed from the gut. Other cephalosporins given parenterally include cefazolin, cefamandole, cefoxitin, cephaloridine, cephacetrile, cefotaxime, and moxalactam.

DISTRIBUTION

Unlike most cephalosporins, the newer drugs cefotaxime and moxalactam do enter the brain. The concentrations of cefazolin, cefoxitin, and cefamandole reached in the bile are higher than those of other members of the class.

METABOLISM

Cephalothin, cephapirin, and cephacetrile are deacetylated to less active derivatives. Toxic reactions in patients with renal failure are unlikely with these compounds, since excess drug accumulation as a result of decreased renal excretion is prevented by hepatic metabolism. Renal failure requires dosage adjustment for those cephalosporins that are not subjected to hepatic metabolism, however.

EXCRETION

All cephalosporins are excreted by the kidney. Most are excreted after glomerular filtration and active tubular secretion. Probenecid blocks acid secretion and increases the plasma concentration of most cephalosporins. Moxalactam is apparently not secreted by the renal tubule; it has a longer plasma half-life than do others of the class, and its excretion is not blocked by probenecid.

ANTIBACTERIAL SPECTRUM

All cephalosporins are active against a wide variety of gram-negative and gram-positive bacteria. Newer cephalosporins, highly resistant to β-lactamases, have extended spectrums. Cefamandole is more active against gram-negative bacteria than are the others of the class. More *E coli* and *Enterobacter* strains are sensitive to cefamandole than are sensitive to other cephalosporins. Cefoxitin, although generally less active than cefamandole, is more active against *Proteus, Serratia,* and *Bacteroides fragilis.* Cefotaxime and moxalactam are more effective than other cephalosporins against *Enterobacter,* indole-positive *Proteus, Providencia stuartii,* influenza, and *Serratia.*

ADVERSE EFFECTS

Hypersensitivity reactions, eg, rash, fever, urticaria, eosinophilia, and, rarely, anaphylaxis, are the most common adverse effects. Results of a Coombs' test may be positive after large doses of cephalosporins, although hemolysis may not be present. Cephalosporins, particularly cephaloridine, have been associated with renal tubular necrosis. The toxic renal effects of cephaloridine and the aminoglycosides may be additive when the two drugs are used together.

AMINOGLYCOSIDES

The ineffectiveness of penicillin against gram-negative bacteria led to the development of the aminoglycosides. Presently used compounds of the class include gentamicin, tobramycin, kanamycin, streptomycin, neomycin, and the more recently developed drug that is resistant to bacterial enzymes, amikacin. All the drugs in this class consist of three joined amino sugars. Their high polarity determines their distribution; they are poorly absorbed from the gut and do not enter the brain. Therefore, they are all given parenterally except for neomycin, which is used not only topically, but also orally (specifically to decrease bacteria in the bowel). All aminoglycosides share similar pharmacologic and toxicity properties. Aminoglycosides are most active against aerobic, gram-negative bacteria, all inhibit bacterial protein synthesis by an action on the ribosome, and all are ototoxic and nephrotoxic.

ANTIBACTERIAL SPECTRUM

The aminoglycosides are primarily effective against gram-negative bacteria, although they are somewhat active against gram-positive bacteria. The gram-positive enterococci and some streptococci are susceptible to gentamicin and streptomycin, and some staphylococci may be sensitive to gentamicin and tobramycin, although this has not been demonstrated clinically. Most gram-negative strains are more sensitive to gentamicin, tobramycin, and amikacin than to kanamycin; however, *Proteus rettgeri, Providencia stuartii,* and *Herellea vaginicola* may be more sensitive to kanamycin. Tobramycin is more active than other members of the class against *Pseudomonas aeruginosa* and some *Proteus* strains.

MECHANISM OF ACTION

All aminoglycosides produce their antibacterial effects by inhibiting bacterial protein synthesis through an action on the ribosome. Mammalian and bacterial ribosomes are structurally different and can be differentiated by their sedimentation (s) coefficients. Mammalian ribosomes consist of 40s and 60s units joined to form an 80s unit. Bacterial ribosomes consist of 30s and 50s subunits, which, together, form a 70s ribosome. The aminoglycoside antibiotics bind to the bacterial 30s ribosomal subunit and, by an as yet unknown mechanism, inhibit normal bacterial protein synthesis. Regardless of the exact step of protein synthesis prevented by the aminoglycosides, these drugs probably change the three-dimensional shape of the protein, thereby altering its ability to function normally. Some data suggest that this binding prevents polysome formation or causes misreading of the genetic code, resulting in abnormal proteins. The exact mechanism remains obscure, however.

PHARMACOKINETICS

The highly polar aminoglycosides are not absorbed from the GI tract, do not enter the brain, and do not enter cells. Their distribution is, therefore, restricted to the extracellular water. Aminoglycosides are negligibly bound to plasma proteins. High concentrations of drug are found only in the renal cortex, which is presumably related to the nephrotoxicity of this class of drugs. Aminoglycoside administration late in pregnancy may result in considerable fetal accumulation of drug. Plasma half-lives are 2 to 3 hours for all drugs of the class. Because all aminoglycosides are excreted unchanged after glomerular filtration, it is critical to adjust the dosage in patients with renal failure.

ADVERSE EFFECTS

The usefulness of the aminoglycosides is greatly limited by their adverse effects. Ototoxicity is manifested by drug-induced damage to sensory vestibular and cochlear hair cells. Damage progresses from the base of the cochlea, which mediates high frequencies, to the apex, which mediates low frequencies. The degree of ototoxic effects is correlated with the plasma drug concentration. Damage is caused gradually and is potentiated by diuretics. Whether ear damage results solely from an osmotic effect or whether it is due to a direct effect of the aminoglycosides is unclear. Some evidence suggests that a loss of hearing has occurred in babies born to mothers given streptomycin during pregnancy, so possible fetal effects must be considered likely.

The nephrotoxic effects of the aminoglycosides consist of usually reversible acute tubular damage with secondary interstitial damage. Kidney damage also occurs gradually and is more common in patients with high plasma drug concentrations. Neomycin, the most nephrotoxic aminoglycoside, is no longer given systemically. Gentamicin, amikacin, and kanamycin produce nephrotoxic effects in approximately 5% of patients. Tobramycin and streptomycin produce nephrotoxic effects in approximately 1% of patients. The mechanism by which these effects are caused is unknown. Evidence suggests that there may be high concentrations of aminoglycosides in the kidneys of babies whose mothers received these drugs during pregnancy.

Hypersensitivity reactions (eg, rash, fever, and lymph gland enlargement) have been reported. Aminoglycosides also have a curarelike effect on the neuromuscular junction and may cause acute paralysis and apnea, as well as a potentiation of the effects of nondepolarizing neuromuscular junction blockers. Myasthenia gravis patients are sensitive to this effect of aminoglycosides, since their neuromuscular function is already impaired. Apparently, aminoglycosides decrease acetylcholine release and postsynaptic sensitivity to acetylcholine.

ERYTHROMYCIN

A macrolide antibiotic named for its large lactone structure, erythromycin contains two deoxy-sugars. Perhaps the most notable thing about erythromycin is its relative lack of serious adverse effects. Erythromycin is active against a variety of gram-positive bacteria and, depending on the organism, can be bacteriostatic or bacteriocidal. Erythromycin inhibits bacterial protein synthesis by binding to the bacterial 50s ribosomal subunit.

Although effective against many of the same bacteria for which penicillin is used, erythromycin is a second choice after penicillin for most organisms. Erythromycin is presently the drug of choice in patients allergic to penicillin and for the treatment of infection with *Mycoplasma pneumoniae*, Legionnaire's disease, diphtheria, pertussis (whooping cough), tetanus, and *Chlamydia* infections.

ANTIBACTERIAL SPECTRUM

Erythromycin is highly active against gram-positive cocci, including *Streptococcus pyogenes*, group B *Streptococcus*, anaerobic *Streptococcus*, *Streptococcus pneumoniae*, the gram-positive *Bacillus anthracis*, *Clostridium perfringens*, *Corynebacterium diphtheriae*, and *Listeria monocytogenes*. Erythromycin is also active against some gram-negative bacteria: *Neisseria gonorrhoeae*, *Neisseria meningitidis*, *Pasteurella multocida*, *Bordetella pertussis*, some *Bacteroides* strains, *Campylobacter fetus*, *Campylobacter jujuni*, *Legionella micdadei*, *Legionella pneumophila*, *Hemophilus ducreyi* (chancroid), and *Leptotrichia buccalis*. Also susceptible are *Chlamydia trachomatis* (inclusion conjunctivitis and pneumonia), *Mycoplasma pneumoniae*, and *Ureaplasma urealyticum*.

MECHANISM OF ACTION

Macrolide antibiotics, including erythromycin, bind to the bacterial 50s ribosomal subunit and have reduced affinity for the mammalian 60s ribosomal subunit. Erythromycin binds to a site on the 50s unit in such a way that it inhibits translocation of the protein-tRNA chain from the aminoacyl site to the peptidyl site, thereby blocking protein elongation and decreasing the normal synthesis of bacterial proteins. Gram-positive bacteria contain far more erythromycin than do gram-negative bacteria, apparently because diffusion of erythromycin across the more complex gram-negative cell wall by the charged erythromycin molecule is decreased. The fact that the antibacterial activity of erythromycin increases as pH increases is probably due to an increase in the proportion of uncharged erythromycin that can more easily enter the gram-negative bacteria.

PHARMACOKINETICS

Erythromycin is inactivated by gastric juice, but readily absorbed from the gut; therefore it is given orally in a coated tablet or as an ester. The plasma half-life of erythromycin is approximately 90 minutes. Erythromycin distributes widely, including the prostatic fluid, the fetus, and cells. It does not enter the brain. Erythromycin is concentrated in the liver and excreted in the bile. Only a small proportion of administered erythromycin is excreted in the urine.

ADVERSE EFFECTS

Erythromycin rarely produces serious adverse effects. Cholestatic hepatitis is a problem when erythromycin estolate is used. It is reversible, but it resembles acute cholecystitis to such a degree that unnecessary surgery has been performed. Other adverse effects include drug allergy, a reversible increase in SGOT levels, epigastric pain after oral ingestion, pain after intramuscular injection of large doses, and thrombophlebitis after large intravenous doses.

ANTIFUNGAL AND ANTIPROTOZOAL DRUGS

Nystatin

A polyene antibiotic produced by *Streptomyces noursei,* nystatin is poorly absorbed from the GI tract and is, therefore, used topically or for its local effect in the gut. Since nystatin is a large molecule with a large hydrophilic portion, it is not absorbed through the skin or mucous membranes. Nystatin is both fungistatic and fungicidal. Sensitive fungi include *Candida, Cryptococcus, Histoplasma, Trichophyton, Epidermophyton, Blastomyces,* and *Microsporum audouini.* Little resistance develops to nystatin. Nystatin rarely causes adverse effects, although nausea, vomiting, and diarrhea can occur after oral use. It is used for *Candida* infections of skin, mucous membranes, and intestine.

Nystatin is a true ionophore. It interacts with the fungal membrane in such a way that a pore or channel is formed in the membrane through which water and small molecules can travel, resulting in a disruption of cell function.

Miconazole

A broad spectrum antifungal agent, miconazole permeates the fungal cell wall, increases its permeability, and disrupts cell function. Miconazole is used intravaginally to treat vulvovaginalis candidiasis and can cause burning, itching, rash, headache, and pelvic cramps early in the treatment. It is also active against some trichomonads. Little miconazole is found in the blood or urine, and it is considered relatively safe in pregnancy.

Clotrimazole

Structurally related to miconazole and similar in antifungal spectrum and mechanism of action is clotrimazole. It is also active against trichomonads that cause vaginitis. Clotrimazole is considered the drug of choice for trichomoniasis during pregnancy. After vaginal application, some patients report a mild burning sensation, cramps, or skin rash. The sexual partner may experience urethral irritation.

Metronidazole

The drug of choice for vaginitis caused by *Trichomonas vaginalis* or *Gardnerella vaginalis* and for nonspecific vaginitis is metronidazole. It is an orally absorbed, systemically distributed antiprotozoal drug that is directly trichomonacidal. It is metabolized and excreted in the urine, which may be reddish brown in color because of pigmented metabolites. Metronidazole can cause nausea, diarrhea, and cramping, as well as headache and vomiting. A metallic taste is not uncommon. Dizziness, vertigo, and ataxia have been reported. Reactive moniliasis can occur during metronidazole therapy, causing furry tongue, stomatitis, and glossitis. Because metronidazole produces a disulfuramlike effect, consumption of alcohol during metronidazole therapy is to be avoided. Metronidazole has been shown to be carcinogenic in animals; therefore, a course of therapy should last for no more than one week at a time. During pregnancy, clotrimazole is the drug of choice for trichomoniasis, although it is less effective than metronidazole. Concurrent treatment of the sexual partner is important to prevent immediate reinfection.

Metronidazole is converted within sensitive organisms to a reduced form that causes DNA breakage and changes the helical structure of DNA. Metronidazole is believed to produce its antibiotic effects by these actions on DNA.

7

Antineoplastic Drugs

Alkylating Agents
  Nitrogen Mustards
    Mechlorethamine (Nitrogen Mustard)
    Cyclophosphamide
    Melphalan (L-PAM, L-sarcolysin)
    Chlorambucil
  Alkyl Sulfonates: Busulfan
  Nitrosoureas
    Carmustine (BCNU)
    Lomustine (CCNU) and Semustine (Methyl-CCNU)
    Chlorozotocin
Antimetabolites
  Folate Analogs: Methotrexate
  Pyrimidine Analogs
    5-Fluorouracil
    Floxuridine (Fluorodeoxyuridine)
    Cytosine Arabinoside
  Purine Analogs
    Mercaptopurine
    Thioguanine
    Adenine Arabinoside and Fluoroadenine Arabinoside
Antibiotics
  Bleomycin
  Actinomycin D
  Daunorubicin and Doxorubicin
Vinca Alkaloids
  Vinblastine
  Vincristine

The biologic reason that a normal cell becomes a cancer cell remains an enigma and a subject of intensive research. Present data suggest that both exogenous factors, such as chemical carcinogens and some viruses, and presently unknown endogenous factors can induce cellular transformation. Once a cancer cell is present and growing, the immune system seems to play a critical role in determining if the cell is seen as "friend or foe" by the body and, therefore, whether it is to be ignored or destroyed by the body.

Although future treatments of cancer will involve the use of selective antibodies that damage cancer cells preferentially and more highly localized delivery of cytotoxic compounds to cancer cells, present therapy for neoplastic diseases primarily involves surgery, radiation, and systemic cytotoxic drug treatment. The obvious goal of cancer chemotherapy is to kill the cancer cells without affecting the normal cells. Most compounds used presently have very low therapeutic indexes because they are intrinsically toxic to both normal and abnormal cells. The toxic effects of many of these drugs are greatest in rapidly dividing cells; therefore, bone marrow depression and death of intestinal and hair follicle cells are expected and unwanted side-effects of chemotherapy. Presently used chemotherapeutic compounds can be divided into five categories: 1) alkylating agents, 2) antimetabolites, 3) antibiotics, 4) miscellaneous agents, and 5) hormones.

ALKYLATING AGENTS

All alkylating agents have the ability to form covalent bonds between the drug molecule and a nucleophilic target molecule. The target molecules include phosphate, hydroxyl, carboxyl, sulfhydryl, amino, or imidazole groups. Although the alkylating agents can bind with any number of cellular constituents, it is generally believed that the cytotoxicity of these compounds is mediated by the alkylation of guanine residues of DNA. Three mechanisms have been suggested to explain the mutagenic and cytotoxic actions of the alkylating agents:

1. A reactive carbonium ion intermediate of the drug binds to a nitrogen atom of guanine (preferably the N^7 position), forming a quaternary ammonium compound. This quaternary guanine compound is more acidic than the normal tertiary one, and the enol tautomer is favored. Rather than undergoing the normal guanine-cytosine bonding, this guanine compound forms base pairs with thymine, leading to a miscoding of the DNA message.

2. Alkylation of the imidazole ring may render it susceptible to cleavage, resulting in DNA damage.

3. Alkylating agents with two active chains can form cross linkages by forming covalent bonds between one guanine residue of DNA and another, or between one guanine residue of DNA and a non-DNA macromolecule. Covalent linkage of DNA to other DNA chains or cellular constituents would, according to this view, disrupt cellular function.

Unlike many other cytotoxic compounds, alkylating agents do not produce their effects on one particular part of the cellular reproductive cycle; they are cytotoxic at any part of the mitotic cycle. Since alkylating agents block cell division, their predominant effects are on rapidly dividing cells. This action involves not only tumor cells, but also hair follicles, gut mucosal cells, bone marrow, thymus, and germinal epithelium of the testes, and the fetus. Amenorrhea of several months' duration sometimes occurs after therapy with alkylating agents. CNS excitation, nausea, vomiting, and convulsions are adverse effects of all nitrogen mustard alkylating agents. In addition, these compounds are immunosuppressive and decrease the ability of the body's natural defenses to recognize and destroy the tumor cells.

Nitrogen Mustards

MECHLORETHAMINE (NITROGEN MUSTARD)

The first nitrogen mustard compound to be used clinically was mechlorethamine. It is chemically unstable, but this property is used to advantage. Mechlorethamine is highly reactive. Within minutes after intravenous (IV) injection, mechlorethamine reacts with body constituents and no longer circulates in an active form. Therefore, the drug can be delivered selectively by injecting it into the artery that perfuses the target organ. Conversely, other organs can be protected from the drug by interrupting blood flow to them during the injection.

The main adverse effects of mechlorethamine include nausea and vomiting, probably as a result of CNS excitation, and bone marrow suppression. Menstrual and fetal abnormalities can be caused by mechlorethamine, probably because of a toxic effect on egg and fetal cell development, respectively. However, no permanent damage to ovarian function is thought to occur. An additional side-effect is related to the extreme chemical reactivity of mechlorethamine. If injected subcutaneously, it causes severe tissue damage.

Mechlorethamine is used in the treatment of Hodgkin's disease, lymphomas, and carcinomas of breast, ovary, and other tissues. Less highly reactive alkylating agents are often preferable to mechlorethamine, however.

CYCLOPHOSPHAMIDE

The hope that a relatively stable congener of mechlorethamine could be formed by masking the reactive portion of the molecule with a phosphate linkage led to the development of cyclophosphamide. It was envisaged that tumor cells might have higher phosphatase activity than do normal cells and that the inert compound could be converted to a cytotoxin predominantly within the cancer cell. In practice, cyclophosphamide is first converted to hydroxycyclophosphamide by the cytochrome P-450, mixed function oxidase system in the liver. Hydroxycyclophosphamide spontaneously tautomerizes to form aldophosphamide, which is converted within cells to two toxic products, phosphoramide mustard and acrolein. Phosphoramide mustard is probably the active alkylator; acrolein, which is excreted in the urine, is probably responsible for the hemorrhagic cystitis and excessive water retention associated with cyclophosphamide therapy. Unlike mechlorethamine, cyclophosphamide is effective when administered orally, does not cause marked tissue damage (because of its relatively stable nature), and produces fewer CNS excitatory effects and less bone marrow depression; however, damage to hair follicles (leading to reversible hair loss) is greater.

Cyclophosphamide is used widely in cancer chemotherapy, often in combination with other cytotoxic drugs. It is effective in the treatment of multiple myeloma, chronic lymphocytic leukemia, cervical and breast carcinoma, ovarian malignancies, bronchogenic carcinoma, and a wide variety of other tumors. Cyclophosphamide is also used as an immunosuppressant for organ transplantation.

MELPHALAN (L-PAM, L-SARCOLYSIN)

Like cyclophosphamide, melphalan was the product of rational drug design. Melphalan is a congener of mechlorethamine in which the methyl group of mechlorethamine is replaced with phenylalanine. It was hoped that tumor cells that have an increased demand for phenylalanine might take up melphalan selectively. In practice, melphalan does enter cells via a competitive amino acid uptake system, but there is little evidence to suggest that melphalan preferentially enters tumor cells that need phenylalanine to synthesize melanin. Melphalan is also less reactive chemically than mechlorethamine and has a spectrum of actions similar to that of other nitrogen mustards. Melphalan is absorbed after oral administration, metabolized, and excreted in the urine. It causes equal and reversible suppression of granulocyte and platelet formation. Unlike cyclophosphamide, melphalan does not cause hemorrhagic cystitis, since no acrolein is formed.

Melphalan has a broad spectrum of activity against tumors, eg, lymphomas, multiple myeloma, and cancers of the breast and ovary.

CHLORAMBUCIL

The cytotoxic effects of chlorambucil and its mechanism of action are similar to those of other alkylating agents. Of all the clinically used nitrogen mustards, chlorambucil is the slowest acting. Given orally over an extended period, it produces its cytotoxic effects gradually, without causing marked bone marrow depression. At clinically used doses, chlorambucil rarely causes CNS excitation, nausea, or vomiting. Toxic effects of chlorambucil on bone marrow and other rapidly dividing tissue are similar to those of other alkylating agents.

Chlorambucil is the drug of choice for treatment of chronic lymphocytic leukemia and primary macroglobulinemia. It is also effective in the treatment of Hodgkin's disease, lymphomas, and cancer of the breast and ovary.

Alkyl Sulfonates: Busulfan

Busulfan consists of a four-carbon alkyl chain with a methane-sulfonate group at each end. The methane-sulfonate groups form reactive carbonium ions, thus allowing alkylation of DNA. Busulfan is unique in that it produces a relatively selective myelosuppression without marked effects on gastrointestinal (GI) epithelium or lymphoid tissue. Given daily by the oral route, busulfan produces a smooth, long-lasting suppression of white cell production. Bone marrow suppression is not rapidly reversible, and high doses of busulfan can cause bone marrow "burn-out" so that careful monitoring of the blood count is required. Busulfan causes diffuse pulmonary fibrosis and cutaneous hyperpigmentation. In addition, the rapid destruction of killed cells greatly increases plasma uric acid and causes precipitation of renal urate. Therefore, allopurinol is used concurrently to decrease urate synthesis. Nausea, vomiting, diarrhea, amenorrhea, and fetal abnormalities have also been reported.

Busulfan's relatively selective effect on white cell production makes it useful for the treatment of chronic granulocytic leukemia. Busulfan is also effective in treating polycythemia vera and myelofibrosis with myeloid metaplasia, but it is of no use in acute leukemia or in the acute "blastic crisis" of chronic granulocytic leukemia.

Nitrosoureas

Nitrosourea alkylating agents (carmustine, lomustine, semustine, and chlorozotocin) differ from the other alkylating agents in that the nitrosoureas are lipid-soluble and, therefore, effective in treating brain tumors and meningeal leukemias. Nitrosoureas are chemically unstable in aqueous solution and spontaneously form two reactive compounds, a chloroethyldiazohydroxide and a second product containing an isocyanate group. The chloroethyldiazohydroxide gives up its nitrogen atoms to form a reactive carbonium ion that then acts like the nitrogen mustards to alkylate DNA, producing cross linkages and strand breaks. The isocyanate product of nitrosourea decomposition reacts with amine groups of amino acids in carbamoylation reactions. This is thought to inhibit DNA repair and RNA processing, but the alkylation of DNA by the chloroethyldiazohydroxide product is believed to be the main cytotoxic mechanism.

Presently used nitrosoureas have a wide spectrum of antitumor activity, but they produce severe myelosuppression. Recent clinical trials of chlorozotocin, however, suggest that this compound may be as efficacious against tumors as other nitrosoureas, but may not have the same myelosuppressive toxicity.

CARMUSTINE (BCNU)

Carmustine is administered IV because, although it is absorbed from the gut, its metabolism is rapid. Carmustine produces its myelosuppressive effects slowly; maximal effects occur 6 weeks after therapy is initiated. High lipid solubility, a property it has in common with other nitrosoureas, allows penetration of the drug into the brain and CSF. Nausea, vomiting, and flushing of the skin occur shortly (within hours) after injection. Prolonged treatment can cause bone marrow "burnout" or pulmonary fibrosis.

Carmustine has a spectrum of antitumor activity similar to that of other alkylating agents. It is useful in the treatment of Hodgkin's disease, lymphomas, myelomas, and tumors of the breast, GI tract, and kidney. In addition, its ability to reach therapeutic concentrations in the brain and CSF make it useful for treating meningeal leukemia, as well as primary and metastatic brain tumors.

LOMUSTINE (CCNU) AND SEMUSTINE (METHYL-CCNU)

The action, toxicity, and clinical uses of lomustine and its methylated derivative semustine are similar to those of carmustine. The main difference lies in the fact that lomustine and semustine are administered orally. Like carmustine, these other nitrosoureas cause a delayed suppression of the bone marrow.

CHLOROZOTOCIN

A still experimental nitrosourea, chlorozotocin may represent a therapeutic advance. Its toxic effect on bone marrow is less than that of the other nitrosoureas, probably because of decreased alkylation of bone marrow DNA.

ANTIMETABOLITES

Because of a structural similarity to endogenous metabolic substances, antimetabolites inhibit a normal physiological process either competitively or noncompetitively by binding to an active site that normally binds the natural metabolite. Antimetabolites can be cytotoxic to a cell that has an absolute requirement for the metabolite. This group of antineoplastic agents includes antifolates, as well as analogs of the pyrimidines and purines used to synthesize nucleotides.

Folate Analogs: Methotrexate

Folates are ingested as either folic acid (petroylglutamate) or as methylated and reduced congeners of folate that contain a variable number of glutamate molecules. Muscosal cells in the duodenum and jejunum contain a carboxypeptidase that reduces the number of glutamate moieties, allowing transport of a less highly charged molecule. These mucosal cells contain dihydrofolate reductase and methylation capability in order to form methyltetrahydrofolate (CH_3-FH_4) from absorbed folic acid. It is this methylated form of folate that is absorbed into the bloodstream and transported to cells throughout the body.

CH_3-FH_4 enters cells by a carrier-mediated membrane transport system. Once inside cells, glutamate molecules are added to form polyglutamates that, as a result of their increased charge, do not readily diffuse from the cell. This methylated and highly reduced form of folate is the active form that is required in a variety of cellular methylation reactions, including the rate-limiting step in DNA synthesis. One cellular reaction involves the methylation of deoxyuridylate to form thymidylate. This reaction is catalyzed by thymidylate synthetase, requires N^{5-10}-methylene-FH_4 as the methyl donor, and generates dihydrofolate (FH_2). In order for the methylated folate to be regenerated, the dihydrofolate must be reduced to tetrahydrofolate by dihydrofolate reductase. It is this metabolic reaction that is inhibited by antifolates.

Since inhibition of this reaction prevents the formation of the required methylated folate derivatives, normal cell function and multiplication cease. Once this effect is understood, the rationale for folinic acid "rescue" can readily be seen. Once tumor cells have been killed with very high doses of antifolate, normal cells can be rescued before death by injecting folinic acid (citrovorum factor, leucovorin). Folinic acid is a fully active folate (N^5-formyl-FH_4) that can either donate a methyl group or be converted to another methyl-donating folate congener by reactions that do not involve the inhibited enzyme dihydrofolate reductase. Folinic acid is effective in blocking the antifolate-induced damage to GI epithelium and bone marrow cells if it is injected 6 to 36 hours after infusions of antifolate.

Although a number of antifolates have antineoplastic efficacy, none are superior to methotrexate, a drug that has been used clinically for a long period and has predictable and manageable adverse effects. Methotrexate is well absorbed from the gut after small doses, but it is erratically absorbed after large doses. It distributes widely, but does not enter the brain or CSF in therapeutic concentrations. Therefore, intrathecal injections are used to affect tumors of the CNS, even though significant neurotoxic effects can result from this method. Methotrexate is bound to plasma proteins and can be displaced by competitive ligands, eg, sulfonamides, diphenylhydantoin, or salicylates. Since plasma concentrations of methotrexate reflect therapeutic efficacy and toxicity, methotrexate levels can be monitored to evaluate the effect of other drugs or renal insufficiency on the concentration of free and, therefore, biologically active methotrexate. Although methotrexate is excreted by the kidney via glomerular filtration and active tubular secretion, intracellular (active) methotrexate, bound to dihydrofolate reductase, stays in the body much longer than plasma levels suggest.

In normal animals, methotrexate severely damages the proliferating cells of the gut, bone marrow, and fetus. Clinically, methotrexate causes similar effects on gut and bone marrow, but these toxic effects can be minimized by folinic acid "rescue" as described earlier. Cell kill is correlated with both the drug concentration and the duration of drug treatment. Methotrexate induces remissions slowly in leukemia, since the mature cells that cause clinical symptoms are not in a proliferative phase. Therefore, methotrexate is most useful for maintaining the remission induced by a faster acting drug.

Methotrexate is useful in the treatment of acute lymphoblastic leukemia of children, choriocarcinoma, hydatiform mole, chorioadenoma destruens, breast carcinoma, mycosis fungoides, and a number of other carcinomas. In addition, methotrexate is effective in treating severe psoriasis and is used for its immunosuppressive activity in organ transplant cases and in autoimmune inflammatory disorders.

Pyrimidine Analogs

Analogs of pyrimidines (normal constituents of DNA and RNA) that possess antitumor activity include 5-fluorouracil (5-FU), 5-fluoro-2-deoxyuridine (floxuridine), and cytosine arabinoside.

5-FLUOROURACIL

Because 5-FU is erratically absorbed from the gut, it is usually given IV. It is metabolized to active and inactive compounds; only a small proportion of an administered dose is pharmacologically active. Renal excretion of the parent compound is minor (10% to 20%). Unlike methotrexate, 5-FU penetrates the brain and reaches therapeutic concentrations in the brain and CSF. Like other antineoplastic agents, 5-FU produces its main toxic effects on the proliferative cells of the bone marrow and GI epithelium. 5-FU reliably produces nausea, stomatitis, and diarrhea, and these effects indicate than an effective dose has been administered.

5-FU must be metabolized by the body in order to exert its antineoplastic effects. There are a variety of possible reactions, but the important ones involve the formation of 5-fluorouridine triphosphate (FUTP) and 5-fluoro-deoxyuridine monophosphate (FdUMP). FUTP is incorporated into RNA, resulting in abnormal RNA and impaired protein synthesis. FdUMP binds to the enzyme thymidylate synthetase. FdUMP and N^{5-10}-methylene tetrahydrofolate form a covalently bound complex with thymidylate synthetase that inactivates the enzyme and decreases the synthesis of deoxythymidine triphosphate. Since deoxythymidine triphosphate is one of the four bases of DNA, synthesis of DNA ceases. The role of FUTP incorporation into RNA in the cytotoxic effects of 5-FU is unclear. Some evidence suggests that both effects of these two 5-FU analogs (FdUMP and FUTP) are important antineoplastic effects of 5-FU.

5-FU is useful in the treatment of GI and breast carcinomas; hepatomas; and ovarian, cervical, and other cancers. It is also useful topically for premalignant keratoses and superficial basal cell carcinoma.

FLOXURIDINE (FLUORODEOXYURIDINE)

The effects of floxuridine are similar to those of 5-FU, since floxuridine is converted in a single step by thymidine kinase to FdUMP, the inhibitor of thymidylate synthetase produced in a series of steps from 5-FU. Floxuridine is also a substrate for thymidine phosphorylase, which converts floxuridine to 5-FU. 5-FU formed from floxuridine undergoes the same reactions undergone by administered 5-FU. Floxuridine is not converted to FUTP (as is 5-FU), however, and does not affect RNA synthesis.

CYTOSINE ARABINOSIDE

Because cytosine arabinoside is poorly absorbed from the gut, it is given by the IV route. After IV injection, it is distributed throughout the total body water and is no longer measurable in plasma 20 minutes after injection. The majority of excreted drug is in the inactive form of arabinosyl uracil, which is produced by the liver, plasma, and peripheral granulocytes. Like 5-FU, cytosine arabinoside penetrates into the brain and CSF. Rapid inactivation of cytosine arabinoside by cytidine deaminase usually necessitates giving cytosine arabinoside by continuous infusion. Like other antimetabolites, the main toxic effects of cytosine arabinoside are myelosuppression and damage to GI epithelium. Cytosine arabinoside is also used intrathecally, since a low deamination rate in CSF provides high drug concentrations for prolonged periods.

Cytosine arabinoside differs from deoxycytidine (the natural precursor of deoxycytidine triphosphate [dCTP]) in the presence of a hydroxyl group in the β, rather than the normal α position of the 2' carbon atom. Since it lacks an oxygen molecule in the α position, it is recognized by the cell to be a deoxy form that can be converted to its active triphosphate form. Therefore, cytosine arabinoside is converted to cytidine triphosphate arabinoside (ara-CTP), which competes with normal deoxycytidine triphosphate for the enzyme DNA polymerase and, therefore, inhibits DNA replication. Cytosine arabinoside is also incorporated into DNA and RNA in the form of cytidine triphosphate arabinoside. The effects of cytosine arabinoside on DNA replication and its incorporation into RNA are believed to explain the cytotoxicity of cytosine arabinoside. Incorporation of cytidine triphosphate arabinoside into DNA may be a less significant effect.

Cytosine arabinoside is highly effective in producing remissions in patients with acute myeloblastic leukemia and is the current drug of choice for this disease. It is also effective against the "blastic crisis" of chronic granulocytic leukemia and acute lymphoblastic leukemia. Its rapid inactivation makes it less useful than other similar drugs for most slowly growing cancers.

Purine Analogs

As a class of drugs, purine analogs include the immunosuppressant drug azathioprine; the antiviral agent ara-adenine; allopurinol, which is used in treating gout; and the anticancer agents mercaptopurine, thioguanine, and fluoro-adenine arabinoside.

MERCAPTOPURINE

Readily absorbed from the GI tract, mercaptopurine is metabolized by the liver; its metabolites are excreted in the urine. One metabolic process involves methylation of the sulfhydryl group of mercaptopurine. The other major metabolic process is catalyzed by the enzyme xanthine oxidase. The amount of available, pharmacologically active mercaptopurine is largely determined by the rate at which mercaptopurine is metabolized by xanthine oxidase; therefore, the xanthine oxidase inhibitor allopurinol greatly increases the potency of mercaptopurine, although its efficacy and therapeutic index are unaffected. When allopurinol is used to prevent the hyperuricemia and resulting renal damage that can follow a large cell kill, the dose of concomitantly administered mercaptopurine must be reduced. When used for the treatment of leukemias, mercaptopurine decreases the total leukocyte count, beginning 1 to 4 weeks after therapy is initiated. The main adverse effect of mercaptopurine is bone marrow depression. Unlike the pyrimidine analogs (5-FU, cytosine arabinoside), antipurines cause less stomatitis and diarrhea; however, nausea and vomiting are not rare. Mercaptopurine also causes a reversible jaundicelike state.

Nucleotides and their precursors serve so many cellular functions that it is often exceedingly difficult to determine which one of the many effects produced by a nucleotide analog is the one responsible for a given effect. This is the case for the antineoplastic effect of the purine analogs. The presently favored view is that mercaptopurine itself is inactive and must be converted by hypoxanthine-guanine phosphoribosyltransferase to 6-thioinosine-5'-phosphate. It is believed that this sulfur-containing monophosphate nucleotide inhibits the first step of purine synthesis by mimicking the feedback inhibitory effect normally produced by the natural nucleotides. This is thought to involve the inhibition of phosphoribosyl-pyrophosphate-amino-transferase, the enzyme that catalyzes the formation of ribosylamine-5-phosphate. Although mercaptopurine can be incorporated into DNA, which may result in defective cell replication, it is unknown if this property is also responsible for the antitumor effects of mercaptopurine.

Mercaptopurine is primarily useful in the treatment of acute leukemias, eg, lymphoblastic leukemia and chronic granulocytic leukemia. It is also an immunosuppressant effective in transplant patients and useful in the treatment of autoimmune diseases.

THIOGUANINE

Because thioguanine is erratically absorbed from the gut, it is given IV. Unlike mercaptopurine, thioguanine itself is not significantly metabolized by xanthine oxidase, and concurrent administration of allopurinol does not necessitate a reduction in thioguanine dosage. The main metabolic reaction is methylation of the sulfur group of thioguanine, which leads to the ultimate removal and excretion in the urine of inorganic sulfur. Other properties and adverse effects of thioguanine are similar to those of mercaptopurine.

The exact mechanism by which thioguanine exerts cytotoxic effects is unclear. However, thioguanine is converted, in a reaction analogous to that described for mercaptopurine, to 6-thioguanosine-5'-phosphate (6TGMP) by hypoxanthine-guanine phosphoribosyltransferase. It is believed that 6TGMP also feedback-inhibits the first step of purine synthesis and, by so doing, blocks the synthesis of nucleotides necessary for normal cell function.

Thioguanine is used, in combination with cytosine arabinoside, in the treatment of acute granulocytic leukemia. It is also an effective immunosuppressant useful in therapy for transplant patients and treatment of autoimmune disorders.

ADENINE ARABINOSIDE AND FLUOROADENINE ARABINOSIDE

The arabinosyl congener of adenine is an effective antitumor compound when converted to the triphosphate (in a reaction analogous to that which activates cytosine arabinoside). It is rapidly deaminated by adenosine deaminase, however, which has led to the idea of concurrent use of adenine arabinoside and a deaminase inhibitor (presently under study). Fluoroadenine arabinoside, a new compound also under study, is resistant to deamination and may become useful in the future.

ANTIBIOTICS

Bleomycin

The bleomycins are a class of unusual compounds of complex structure. Clinically used bleomycin is a mixture of bleomycin A_2 and B_2, which differ only in their terminal moieties. It is administered parenterally and is found in high concentrations in skin and lung, the sites of bleomycin toxic effects. The elimination half-life is 2 to 9 hours. Most of the drug is excreted in the urine; the parent molecule and the half-life is prolonged in patients with renal impairment. Bleomycin not only has a wide spectrum of antitumor activity, but also produces minimal bone marrow depression, immunosuppression, or damage to GI epithelium. This is a clear difference between bleomycin and most other antineoplastic drugs.

The main toxic effects caused by bleomycin involve skin reactions. Nearly half of the patients receiving bleomycin develop erythema, induration, peeling of the skin over the palms and joints, and hyperpigmentation. The main adverse effect of bleomycin is its pulmonary effect, however. Bleomycin causes a pneumonitis leading to interstitial fibrosis that can be fatal. The pulmonary syndrome consists of cough, dyspnea, and the appearance of bibasilar pulmonary infiltrates. Interstitial fibrosis decreases oxygen diffusion capacity, particularly among elderly patients. These effects are, of course, complicated by existing pulmonary diseases in which oxygen diffusion is already impaired, eg, emphysema.

Bleomycin produces cytotoxic effects by a unique mechanism. The bleomycin molecule consists of an S-peptide portion and an iron-binding portion. The S-peptide portion of the molecule binds to guanine bases of DNA. The iron (Fe^{2+}) becomes oxidized to Fe^{3+}, and the liberated electron combines with oxygen or hydroxyl groups to produce free radicals. It is envisaged that the generated radicals attack the glycosidic linkages between DNA bases, since free bases are liberated by bleomycin. In this way, bleomycin causes multiple DNA breaks, resulting in impaired cell function and cell death.

Bleomycin seems to act preferentially at the premitotic or mitotic phases, although this remains a subject of controversy. The possibility that bleomycin may be more effective during some stages of the cell cycle than others has led to the use of bleomycin infusion in the hope of improving the cell kill. A bleomycin hydrolase is present in most tissues except for skin and lung, and bleomycin's toxic effects on skin and lung may be due to the high drug concentration found in these tissues as a result of decreased metabolism.

Bleomycin is active against a variety of tumors, including squamous cell carcinomas of the head, neck, esophagus, and skin, as well as tumors of the cervix, vulva, testicles, and penis. It is also active against Hodgkin's disease and a variety of lymphomas.

Actinomycin D

Although actinomycin D is absorbed after oral administration, parenteral injection is far more effective. Actinomycin D distributes widely, is not metabolized, and is excreted into the bile and urine. All rapidly dividing cells are inhibited by actinomycin D, and this leads to the adverse effects typical of many antitumor drugs, ie, bone marrow depression and GI epithelial toxic effects. An interesting and enigmatic effect of actinomycin D involves a synergistic toxic effect on the skin and the GI tract when administration of the drug is combined with x-ray irradiation. There seems to be synergism even when actinomycin D is given months after irradiation.

The phenoxazone ring of actinomycin D inserts perpendicularly into the long axis of the DNA double helix. The adjacent polypeptide chains of actinomycin D bind to deoxyguanosine residues of DNA, and these reactions result in a highly stable complex of actinomycin D and DNA. RNA polymerases are unable to transcribe the DNA message, and protein synthesis is blocked. Actinomycin D is believed to produce its cytotoxic effects in normal and neoplastic cells by this blockade of DNA transcription.

Actinomycin D is used in the treatment of Wilms' tumor and rhabdomyosarcoma, Ewing's tumor, Kaposi's sarcoma, and other soft tissue sarcoma. Gestational choriocarcinoma is also effectively treated with actinomycin D.

Daunorubicin and Doxorubicin

Both daunorubicin and doxorubicin are anthracycline antibiotics; they differ from each other by only a single hydroxyl group. This seemingly minor molecular difference confers an important difference in pharmacologic activity. Whereas daunorubicin is used primarily in treating acute leukemias, doxorubicin is also highly active against a variety of other tumors. Both daunorubicin and doxorubicin are given IV. They do not appear to cross the blood-brain barrier. Because the drugs are metabolized primarily by the liver, a major determinant of the dose administered is liver, not renal, function. In addition to their antineoplastic effects, daunorubicin and doxorubicin cause bone marrow depression, stomatitis, alopecia, and GI disturbances, as well as extremely severe tissue damage after extravasation. In addition, anthracyclines can cause an often fatal cardiomyopathy; it is related to dose, however, so that risk can be minimized by considering dosage carefully. The cardiomyopathy consists of arrhythmias, tachycardia, dyspnea, hypotension, and congestive heart failure that is not responsive to digitalis.

The exact mechanism by which these anthracyclines cause cytotoxic effects is unclear. The available evidence suggests a number of inhibitory actions on cell function. First, both daunorubicin and doxorubicin intercalate between DNA strands. This binding to DNA inhibits DNA and RNA synthesis, leading to inhibitory effects on cell division and growth. Second, these compounds cause DNA breaks and inhibit DNA repair mechanisms. Some evidence suggests that the anthracycline-induced DNA breakage results from a change in three-dimensional DNA structure that renders it susceptible to abnormal enzymatic cleavage. Other evidence suggests that anthracyclines are converted to free radicals by a membrane-associated P-450 reductase and that the DNA breaks occur as a result of radical attack. It has been suggested that the antitumor effects of anthracyclines may be mediated by DNA intercalation and that the toxic effects on the heart may be due primarily to free radical attack. Although unproved, this theory implies that it may be possible to develop anthracyclines that intercalate DNA, but are less susceptible to radical formation. If so, antitumor compounds without significant cardiomyopathic activity may be developed. Third, anthracyclines bind to membrane lipids, eg, cardiolipin and the protein spectrin. Whether these compounds produce their antitumor and cardiotoxic effects by one or a combination of mechanisms remains to be determined.

Daunorubicin is used primarily for the treatment of acute lymphocytic and myelocytic leukemias and malignant lymphomas. Doxorubicin is also useful against a variety of solid tumors. Given with cis-platinum, doxorubicin is effective against ovarian carcinoma; with prednisone, cyclophosphamide, vincristine, and bleomycin, it is effective against lymphomas. It is also useful in the treatment of oat cell carcinoma, metastatic breast adenocarcinoma, metastatic thyroid carcinoma, bronchogenic carcinoma, and carcinomas of testes, prostate, head, neck, endometrium, and cervix.

VINCA ALKALOIDS

The clinically used drugs vinblastine and vincristine, as well as the recently developed analog vindesine (deacetylvinblastine), are the vinca alkaloids.

Vinblastine

Since extreme tissue irritation and damage are caused by direct exposure to vinblastine solution, it is injected directly into an IV infusion tube or into the vein by means of a needle that was not used to fill the syringe. After injection, the concentration of vinblastine declines in plasma biphasically, with half-lives of 4.5 and 190 minutes. A third kinetic phase of 20 hours has been reported. Vinblastine is metabolized by the liver, and the metabolites are excreted in the bile. Therefore, vinblastine dosage must be decreased in patients with liver damage. A minimal amount of vinblastine is excreted by the kidney. The main toxic effects of vinblastine are bone marrow suppression and CNS changes. The latter effects are characterized by a loss of deep tendon reflexes, paresthesias of the fingers and extremities, headache, psychosis, and convulsions. Altered autonomic function is characterized by constipation, dry mouth, an inability to urinate, and ileal paralysis, all likely signs of decreased parasympathetic cholinergic tone.

Vinblastine is believed to produce its cytotoxic effects by stopping mitosis in metaphase as a result of binding to the cellular protein tubulin, a ubiquitous protein that plays a role in chromosome migration during mitosis, the maintenance of cell shape and structure, and the transport of cellular constituents from one part of the cell to another. When vinblastine binds to tubulin, crystals of vinblastine and tubulin are formed in equimolar amounts. It is likely that vinca alkaloids produce their cytotoxic effects and many of the CNS changes by a disruption of cellular tubulin.

Vinblastine is used clinically in the treatment of testicular tumors; lymphomas, including Hodgkin's disease; neuroblastoma; choriocarcinoma; and carcinoma of the breast.

Vincristine

In terms of its mechanism of action and clinical effects, vincristine is similar to vinblastine. The main differences are that vincristine is excreted more rapidly than is vinblastine, causes less myelosuppression than does vinblastine, and is more effective against lymphoblastic leukemia than is vinblastine. Its main adverse effects are the same CNS effects produced by vinblastine.

MISCELLANEOUS DRUGS

Inorganic Platinum Complexes

When electrical current is passed between platinum electrodes, antibacterial compounds are produced in the solution. These compounds are chloride and ammonia-containing platinum compounds. The most active of these is cis(II)-diamminedichloroplatinum (cis-platinum), which is simply a single platinum atom to which are attached two chloride atoms and two ammonia groups in the cis configuration. Trans-platinum, in which the two ammonia groups are in the trans configuration, is without antitumor activity.

Cis-platinum is given IV because it is not absorbed from the gut. More than 90% of cis-platinum in blood is bound to plasma proteins. The initial plasma half-life after injection is approximately 30 minutes. The plasma elimination half-life is 2.5 to 3 days, probably because so much of the drug is bound covalently to plasma and tissue proteins. Cis-platinum is excreted in the urine after glomerular filtration and, to an unknown extent, in the bile. It enters cells by diffusion, but does not readily cross the blood-brain barrier. The adverse effects of cis-platinum involve primarily the kidney and the ear. Renal damage can be minimized by prior hydration and diuresis. Without prehydration, renal toxic effects occur in 30% of patients and are manifested by distal tubular necrosis. Effects on the ear consist of tinnitus and loss of high frequencies. Cis-platinum also causes nausea and vomiting, moderate myelosuppression, sensory neuropathy, and hypersensitivity reactions.

After entry into cells, the two chloride groups of cis-platinum are hydrolyzed, leaving a reactive platinum intermediate that is capable of forming two bonds. This reactive platinum molecule is analogous to the reactive carbonium ion intermediate of the alkylating agents. Like the nitrogen mustards, cis-platinum binds to the N^7 position of guanine and the N^3 position of cytosine in DNA. Resulting cross links between DNA strands are believed to block DNA synthesis and lead to cell death.

Cis-platinum is effective alone or in combination against testicular tumors and carcinomas of the ovary, bladder, head, neck, and endometrium.

Hydroxyurea

Not only is hydroxyurea readily absorbed after oral administration, but also it is largely eliminated from the body within 1 day. It is excreted primarily in the urine. In addition to its antineoplastic actions, hydroxyurea causes bone marrow suppression, consisting of leukopenia, megaloblastic anemia, and thrombocytopenia. Skin and GI reactions, as well as alopecia, are not uncommon adverse effects of hydroxyurea.

Hydroxyurea is believed to produce its cytotoxic effects by inhibiting the enzyme ribonucleoside diphosphate reductase, which catalyzes the conversion of ribonucleotides to deoxyribonucleotides. This reaction is believed to be a rate-limiting step for DNA synthesis.

Hydroxyurea is effective against chronic granulocytic leukemia, metastatic melanoma, and uterine-cervical carcinoma.

Hexamethylmelamine and Pentamethylmelamine

Hexamethylmelamine is given orally, because it is poorly soluble in aqueous solution. It is metabolized by the liver and has a plasma half-life of 5 to 10 hours. During a course of therapy, hexamethylmelamine causes nausea and vomiting increasingly. These are the main adverse effects limiting its usefulness. Hexamethylmelamine has mild effects on bone marrow function and may produce neurotoxic effects characterized by mood changes, hallucinations, peripheral neuropathy, and convulsions. Pentamethylmelamine has one less methyl group than does hexamethylmelamine. It is, therefore, more water-soluble and can be given by the IV route.

The exact antineoplastic mechanism of the methylmelamines is unknown. These compounds are *N*-demethylated by the liver, and this reaction yields formaldehyde, which is only weakly cytotoxic. Since both hexamethylmelamine and pentamethylmelamine must undergo hepatic metabolism to produce their cytotoxic effects, it seems likely that a reactive intermediate is formed and that this intermediate binds to cellular constituents much as the alkylating agents do. This mechanism remains conjectural.

Hexamethylmelamine and pentamethylmelamine are used in the treatment of lymphomas, small cell cancer of the lung, and carcinomas of the breast and ovary.

HORMONES AND HORMONE ANTAGONISTS

A variety of tissues in the body are targets of steroid sex hormones and require the presence of these hormones for optimal growth. Because neoplastic cells that originate from these tissues retain their susceptibility to influence by these hormones, three treatments are possible:

1. The tissues that produce the hormones that promote cancer growth can be removed, eg, orchiectomy, oophorectomy, adrenalectomy, and hypophysectomy.
2. A hormone that inhibits cell growth can be used.
3. A receptor antagonist of a growth-promoting hormone can be given.

It is thought that all steroid hormones produce cellular changes by a similar mechanism. Cells that are targets for the actions of a steroid hormone possess a cytoplasmic steroid receptor. Steroids are highly lipid-soluble and probably enter all cells by passive diffusion. Whether a cell responds to a steroid hormone that has entered it probably depends on whether the cell possesses a cytoplasmic receptor for that hormone. Once the steroid has combined with its cytoplasmic receptor, the complex is translocated to the nucleus. The complex binds to DNA, and there is a resulting increase in RNA and protein synthesis. The exact mechanism by which the steroid and receptor complex increase RNA synthesis remains to be elucidated, as do the exact identities and functions of the synthesized proteins.

Estrogens

Clinically used and orally active estrogens include diethylstilbestrol, conjugated estrogens, and ethinyl estradiol. The antitumor effects of estrogens are manifested slowly (over weeks) and involve regression of neoplasms in the lymph nodes, skin, and breast. Estrogens are commonly used for the treatment of postmenopausal breast cancer. Adverse effects of diethylstilbestrol include loss of appetite, nausea, and vomiting. Effects of all estrogens include incontinence, pigmentation of the nipples, sodium and water retention, and increased libido. The high doses of estrogens used against neoplasms produce far higher concentrations than those that occur physiologically. The mechanism by which high-dose estrogen therapy inhibits postmenopausal neoplastic cell growth is unknown, but it appears to be mediated by the cytoplasmic estrogen receptor.

Progestational Agents

High doses of progestins have been used successfully on an empirical basis for the treatment of breast and endometrial carcinoma. Compounds used include medroxyprogesterone acetate, megestrol acetate, and hydroxyprogesterone. The sensitivity of endometrial cancer to progestins depends on the type of tumor. Highly differentiated endometrial cancer cells are more responsive to progestins than are poorly differentiated tumors; this difference appears to be related to the higher density of progesterone receptors in highly differentiated cells. Although the mechanism by which high-dose progestin therapy produces neoplastic regression is unknown, progestins may bind to progesterone or testosterone, but not estrogen, receptors to produce their effects.

Androgens

The orally active androgens fluoxymesterone and calusterone, and the parenterally administered testosterone proprionate and dromostanolone proprionate are commonly used as antineoplastic drugs. The mechanism by which androgens produce antineoplastic effects in postmenopausal women is unknown, but it is thought to be mediated by cytoplasmic androgen receptors. The main adverse effects of androgen therapy are virilization, increased libido, and erythrocytosis.

Antiestrogens: Tamoxifen

An orally active estrogen receptor antagonist, tamoxifen is replacing other hormonal therapies in postmenopausal patients with estrogen receptor protein-positive tumors. After absorption, the concentration of tamoxifen declines in the plasma biphasically. The initial half-life is 7 to 14 hours, but the terminal elimination phase half-life is greater than 7 days. Tamoxifen produces a "flare" reaction characterized by bone pain and hypercalcemia, which indicates that an antitumor effect will follow. Adverse effects are rare, but they include hot flashes, nausea, and vomiting.

Tamoxifen is a cytoplasmic estrogen receptor antagonist that binds to the receptor. The exact mechanism by which tamoxifen produces antitumor effects is unknown. The decreased estrogenic response is likely to be the result of both decreased receptor availability and the translocation of an abnormal ligand-receptor complex into the nucleus. The fact that tamoxifen is most effective in postmenopausal women with estrogen receptor protein-positive tumors suggests that the estrogen receptor mediates tamoxifen's antitumor effects.

Tamoxifen is useful in the treatment of advanced metastatic breast cancer.

8

Therapeutic Principles

PRESCRIPTION ORDER WRITING

Once a patient has been examined, the appropriate drug, the dosage, and the duration of therapy must be determined and conveyed to both the pharmacist and the patient. It is ironic that, after a clinical evaluation requiring considerable time and judgment, the incorrect choice of a drug or the refusal of the patient to take the drug can turn the entire process into a pointless exercise. If therapy is to be successful, the physician must be able not only to prescribe the correct treatment, but also to communicate effectively with the pharmacist and the patient.

Basic Rules

LANGUAGE

A prescription should be written entirely in grammatically correct English, with no Latin abbreviations, eg, b.i.d. or q.i.d. In the age of the quasi-enlightened consumer, a coded message can be misinterpreted as a means of concealing information from the patient. In addition, although pharmacists are trained to read prescriptions with Latin abbreviations, physicians are generally not properly trained in pharmacy notation, and this can lead to ineffective communication and misunderstanding. Latin phrases no longer serve a useful purpose and can be easily misunderstood when written unclearly.

CHOICE OF DRUG NAME

Ideally, drug names should be written as their nonproprietary or generic names. For example, the benzodiazepine diazepam should be written as diazepam, not as Valium. The drug itself is diazepam in any country, at any time. While the drug is under patent protection, the two names are synonymous. After patent protection ends, this is no longer the case. Since many state legislatures permit or even mandate generic drug substitution, the generic name should be used routinely. Legislative action is being considered that might require the use of generic prescription in some instances, and the physician should be aware of new developments and local regulations.

The advantage of using generic drug names is that it allows the pharmacist to substitute a cheaper form of the same drug when he or she knows that different brands of the same chemical have similar bioavailability. Conversely, the advantage of using a specific trade name is that some generic preparations may have known bioavailability problems. It is best to write the generic name followed by the trade name in parentheses if the specific brand of the drug has known advantages.

Although prescriptions should obviously be written legibly, this is not a universal practice. The physician must, therefore, be aware that the trade names of many drugs sound alike or look alike and that the prescription order form is a legal document for which the physician could be held responsible should a dangerous misunderstanding occur.

SYSTEMS OF WEIGHTS AND MEASURES

The metric system should be used in all cases. Table 8–1 gives the metric equivalents of the apothecary weights and measures.

Order Form

The obvious purpose of a prescription order form is to tell the pharmacist what to dispense and what to put on the label of the drug container. A prescription order form must include the date the prescription was written and the name of the patient (Fig 8–1). The first name should be used, since different members of the family should be able to determine which medicine belongs to which member

Table 8–1. *Metric Equivalents of Apothecary Weights and Measures*

1 milligram	1/65 grains
1 gram	15.43 grains
1 kilogram	2.20 pounds
1 milliliter	16.23 minims
1 grain	65 milligrams
1 ounce	31.1 grams
1 minim	0.062 milliliters
1 fluid ounce	29.57 milliliters
1 pint (U.S.)	473.2 milliliters
1 quart (U.S.)	946.4 milliliters

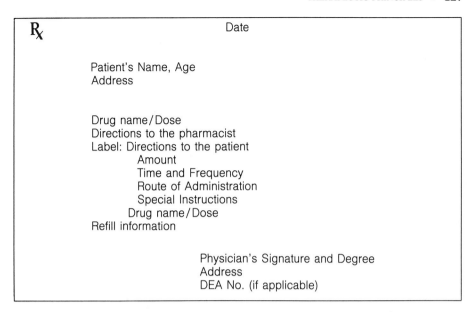

Fig 8–1. *Prescription order form.*

of the family. The age should also be included, as should the address. The full name and address is required by law for all Schedule II drugs.

The inscription is the part of the prescription that lists the drug name and the dose to be dispensed. The subscription directs the pharmacist to dispense a particular number of tablets or capsules, or volume of liquid. The amount of drug prescribed at one time must be based on the mental state of the patient, the illicit value of the drug, and the intrinsic toxicity of the drug. There is little risk of drug abuse or overdose with penicillin; however, the total prescribed amount of drug that a depressed patient might use to commit suicide should obviously not be a lethal dose.

The signature of the prescription (not the physician's signature) tells the pharmacist what to write on the label. It should be preceded by the word *label.* The signature of the prescription is then followed by the refill information. Prescriptions for Schedule II drugs cannot be refilled. Other drugs can be refilled up to five times during the six-month period after the date the prescription was written. Whether a prescription is to be refilled is under the discretion of the physician, and this information must be written in the prescription, eg, do not refill, refill 3 times, refill 5 times. The physician's signature, including the appropriate professional degree, follows this information. For Schedule II drugs, the physician's address and Drug Enforcement Agency (DEA) number must be included. The physician's signature must be in ink or indelible pencil.

It has already been stated that the nonproprietary or generic name of a drug should be used, followed by the proprietary or trade name if a particular product is to be dispensed. After the name of the drug, the dosage is written in metric measurements. This can be done in two ways. A tablet containing 50 mg drug can be written as 50 mg, or the vertical decimal line can be used if a number of drugs are prescribed. For example, if 10 mg drug x, 1 g drug y, and 1 mg drug z are prescribed as a mixture, the prescription would be written as shown in Figure 8–2. The decimal line denotes the location of the decimal point. When a decimal line is used, the drug quantities are understood to be in grams and milliliters. The signature of the prescription, which conveys the physician's instructions to the patient, should describe how the drug is to be used, eg, take . . . , apply . . . , insert. . . . It also includes the amount to be used, how often, and when, eg, take 2 tablets at 12 noon and before bed. The purpose of the medication should be included, unless including it would embarrass the patient. In such a case, verbal or written instructions should be given directly to the patient. The signature of the prescription should list the drug and dosage after the instructions for use in case of suspected overdose, drug allergy, or future confusion when, long after a drug was prescribed, the patient or family members do not remember what was in an undiscarded vial.

PATIENT COMPLIANCE

There are a number of weak links in the therapeutic process. One that often undermines effective pharmacologic therapy is poor patient compliance. There are a bewildering number of reasons that a patient fails to take a drug as prescribed. This subject is more a psychologic than a pharmacologic one, since noncompliance is often a matter of a patient's motives. Although the number of reasons for noncompliance may approach the number of noncompliant patients, some main determinants of noncompliance have been noted in numerous studies.

Fig 8–2. *Sample prescription written in two ways to illustrate the use of the metric line.*

Drug x	10 mg		0	01
Drug y	1 g	or	1	0
Drug z	1 mg		0	001

Make 20 doses and place in 20 capsules.
Label: Take 1 capsule at 8:00 AM, 12 noon, and 4:00 PM for back pain.
Drugs x, y, and z.

The Nature of the Illness

Misery and fear are effective motivators for compliance. If a patient is informed that an extremely painful cough is due to pneumonia, there is a good chance that the patient will follow the prescribed antibiotic therapy assiduously. Conversely, if a patient is found on routine physical examination to have moderate hypertension (asymptomatic), the adverse effects of any antihypertensive therapy might be enough to discourage compliance if the patient is not fully convinced of the need for treatment. These two examples highlight the need for effective communication between physician and patient. If the patient with pneumonia is not told why it is important to complete a course of antibiotic therapy, the patient is likely to stop taking the drug as soon as he or she feels well, thereby risking reinfection. Similarly, the hypertensive patient must be made to realize that a life-threatening illness may exist, despite the fact that the patient has felt unwell only since beginning antihypertensive therapy. In the case of this asymptomatic patient, fear of future consequences may be the most important factor for compliance. Sometimes, the nature of the illness itself can affect compliance; for example, a paranoid schizophrenic may think the drug is a poison, or a depressed patient may be too depressed to get out of bed, let alone follow a prescribed regimen.

The Patient

Obviously, some elderly patients fail to take drugs as prescribed because of forgetfulness. Children fail to comply because they understand neither the need for the drug nor the instructions; therefore, children rely on parental guidance. The family situation in which a patient lives also affects compliance. Numerous studies have shown that patients having concerned spouses, parents, or friends are far more compliant than those living alone. Since a concerned spouse or parent has the incentive of wanting to see the patient well without having to suffer the disincentive of adverse side-effects, a concerned family member is obviously a strong force for compliance.

Additional factors affecting compliance include the obvious problem of a language barrier. Individuals whose native language is not English may routinely answer in the affirmative when asked if they understand what has just been said; however, the physician must question such a patient to ensure that he or she understands exactly when the medication is to be taken, what it is supposed to do, and what adverse effects are to be expected. Finally, a psychoanalytic approach has been used to explain patient compliance. According to this view, tablets and capsules resemble breasts and penises, respectively, and patients' attitudes toward the latter may influence their use of the former. Perhaps the reader should regard this psychoanalytic view of patient compliance as somewhat speculative.

The Medication

For patients not covered by a prescription plan, the cost of the medication can result in failure to have a prescription filled. If a patient with an asymptomatic illness is instructed to take an expensive drug for a long period, the cost may favor noncompliance.

Adverse effects are a major cause of noncompliance. Patients routinely weigh the benefit versus cost (in terms of money as well as discomfort) of any drug treatment. For a patient suffering moderate pain, the constipating effect of codeine, for example, may lead to noncompliance. In this case, noncompliance would not be dangerous, since the patient can best decide which pain, eg, wound or intestinal, he or she prefers to endure. If an illness absolutely requires pharmacologic treatment, however, noncompliance due to adverse effects could be extremely dangerous, and the physician must make clear the serious nature of the illness, inform the patient of the expected side-effects, and discuss the possibility of reducing the dose or changing drugs in the future, if necessary, rather than ceasing to take the drug.

A number of studies have shown that the longer the period of treatment, the more likely a patient is to stop taking the drug. One study showed that there was a positive correlation between the duration of treatment and the degree of noncompliance in pregnant women taking iron. Conversely, for a similar number of patients taking drugs for serious illnesses, no such relationship existed. This suggests that the perceived unimportance of the former therapy may have played a role in noncompliance. Similar results have been shown in studies of patients who feel well and apparently think that continued antibiotic therapy is unnecessary or not worth the bother and expense. In addition, the more complex a regimen, the greater the noncompliance. A decrease in compliance has been reported in a number of studies when the number of drugs taken simultaneously or the number of doses of a single drug increases.

The Physician-Patient Relationship

The attitude of the physician and his or her ability to communicate effectively with the patient are major determinants of the success of drug therapy. One study of compliance among pediatric outpatients showed that compliance was decreased among mothers who perceived the physician as unfriendly or who felt that the physician did not clearly understand the complaint. Compliance is also better when the child is cared for by a familiar physician rather than by rotating staff. Clearly, the reasons that a particular drug has been chosen, how and why it is to be taken, and the expected side-effects should be communicated to the patient. Careful questioning of the patient to determine if the patient understands the instructions and follow-up questioning once drug therapy is under way would greatly improve compliance.

Consequences of Noncompliance

The obvious consequence of noncompliance is that the patient does not receive the beneficial effects of the drug, thereby risking continuation of the condition and worse for serious diseases. Conversely, noncompliance also means that the patient does not suffer from the effects of drugs prescribed in error by the physician. Given the widespread misuse and overuse of prescription drugs, noncompliance cannot be viewed as entirely undesirable.

Detection of the Drug Defaulter

Both subjective and objective methods can be used to identify the drug defaulter. A number of studies have shown that subjective methods are ineffective, however. Fully 83% of parents asked replied that their children were taking penicillin as prescribed, although 92% of urine samples from these children were devoid of antibiotic activity. Furthermore, patients who are noncompliant with one drug may be highly compliant with another. Physicians seem no better than anyone else in predicting which patients are taking drugs as prescribed.

A number of objective means to determine patient compliance have been used, such as adding a marker (eg, phenol red), riboflavin, or stool markers to the drug, but this has little use in routine practice. The most effective method is to ask for a urine sample or take a blood sample without prior notification. Subsequent analysis for the drug itself is obviously the most accurate method to determine if the patient is taking the drug. The possibility of noncompliance should be considered carefully before it is concluded that a particular treatment has been ineffective.

OVER-THE-COUNTER DRUGS

In the minds of many consumers, over-the-counter drugs are freely available because they are safe and can be used without special knowledge. Because of the nature of over-the-counter drug marketing, many consumers do not regard these compounds as "real" drugs and do not include these drugs when asked by a physician what drugs they have been taking. Since diagnostic evaluation is only as valid as the information obtained, it is important to take over-the-counter drugs into account when questioning a patient. Some over-the-counter drugs have important effects. For example, aspirin can prolong labor and postpartum hemorrhage because it inhibits the cyclooxygenase system. Acetaminophen can cause a potentially fatal hepatic necrosis when as few as 15 tablets (6 g) are taken. Vasoconstrictors in nasal decongestant sprays and cold remedies can produce adverse effects in hypertensive patients. Similarly, antacids taken chronically can cause osteomalacia (in the case of aluminum hydroxide gel). All drugs must be taken into account when questioning a patient, giving instructions, or attempting to understand a possible drug interaction.

Appendix

─────────────Appendix A─────────────

BIBLIOGRAPHY

Abramowicz M (ed): *The Medical Letter.* New Rochelle, NY, The Medical Letter Press
   Recent developments in the clinical use of drugs.

Berkowitz RL, Coustan DR, Mochizuki TK: *Handbook for Prescribing Medications during Pregnancy.* Boston, Little, Brown, 1981
   Clinical use of drugs during pregnancy.

Gibaldi M, Prescott L (eds): *Handbook of Clinical Pharmacokinetics.* New York, ADIS Health Science Press, 1983
   Details of the clinical pharmacokinetics of a wide variety of drugs.

Gilman AG, Goodman LS, Gilman A (eds): *The Pharmacological Basis of Therapeutics.* New York, Macmillan, 1980
   Additional information on pharmacology and therapeutics.

Hansten PD: *Drug Interactions.* Philadelphia, Lea & Febiger, 1979
   Additional information on clinical drug interactions.

Harkness R: *OTC Handbook.* Oradell, NJ, Medical Economics, 1983
   Uses and interactions of over-the-counter drugs.

Melmon KL, Morelli HF (eds): *Clinical Pharmacology: Basic Principles in Therapeutics.* New York, Macmillan, 1978
   In-depth information on clinical pharmacology and therapeutic principles.

Physicians' Desk Reference. Oradell, NJ, Medical Economics, 1984
   A compendium of prescription drugs approved for use in the United States, their approved uses, indications, and contraindications.

Appendix B

GLOSSARY OF GENERIC AND TRADE NAMES

acetaminophen	DATRIL, TYLENOL
acetazolamide	DIAMOX
actinomycin D	DACTINOMYCIN
albuterol	PROVENTIL, VENTOLIN
allopurinol	LOPURIN, ZYLOPRIM
amikacin	AMIKIN
amiloride	MIDAMOR
amoxicillin	WYMOX, LAROTID, POLYMOX, TRIMOX
ampicillin	AMCILL, OMNIPEN, POLYCILLIN
bendroflumethiazide	NATURETIN
benzthiazide	AQUATAG, AQUEX, EXNA, HYDREX
bleomycin	BLENOXANE
busulfan	MYLERAN
calusterone	METHOSARB
captopril	CAPOTEN
carbenicillin	GEOPEN
carmustine	BiCNU
cefaclor	CECLOR
cefadroxil	DURICEF, ULTRACEF
cefazolin	ANCEF, KEFZOL
cefotaxime	CLAFORAN
cefoxitin	MEFOXIN
cephalexin	KEFLEX
cephalothin	KEFLIN
cephamandole	MANDOL
cephapirin	CEFADYL

(continued)

GLOSSARY OF GENERIC AND TRADE NAMES (continued)

cephradine	ANSPOR, VELOSEF
chlorambucil	LEUKERAN
chlordiazepoxide	LIBRIUM
chlorothiazide	DIURIL
chlorthalidone	HYGROTON
cinnamedrine	MIDOL
cis-platinum	PLATINOL
clonidine	CATAPRES
clotrimazole	LOTRIMIN, MYCELEX
cloxacillin	TEGOPEN
cyclophosphamide	CYTOXAN
cytosine arabinoside	CYTOSAR-U
daunorubicin	CERUBIDINE
diazepam	VALIUM
diazoxide	HYPERSTAT
dicloxacillin	DYCILL, DYNAPEN, PATHOCIL
diethylstilbestrol	STILPHOSTROL
diflunisal	DOLOBID
dinoprostone (PGE$_2$)	PROSTIN E2
dinoprost tromethamine (PGF$_{2\alpha}$)	PROSTIN F2 ALPHA
diphenoxylate (combination)	DI-ATRO, LOMOTIL, LONOX
doxorubicin	ADRIAMYCIN
dromostanolone	DROLBAN
ergonovine	ERGOTRATE
erythromycin	ILOTYCIN, PEDIAMYCIN
erythromycin estolate	ROBIMYCIN, STATICIN
estrogens, conjugated	PREMARIN, OVEST
ethacrynic acid	EDECRIN
ethinyl estradiol	ESTINYL, FEMINONE
fenoprofen	NALFON
fentanyl	INNOVAR, SUBLIMAZE
floxuridine	FUDR
5-fluorouracil	ADRUCIL, FLUOROURACIL
fluoxymesterone	ANDROID-F, HALOTESTIN

(continued)

GLOSSARY OF GENERIC AND TRADE NAMES (continued)

flurazepam	DALMANE
furosemide	LASIX
gentamicin	GARAMYCIN
guanethidine	ISMELIN, ESIMIL
hetacillin	VERSAPEN
hexobarbital	SOMBULEX
hydralazine	APRESOLINE
hydrochlorothiazide	HydroDIURIL
hydrocodone	HYCODAN
hydroflumethiazide	DIUCARDIN, SALURON
hydromorphone	DILAUDID
hydroxyprogesterone	DELALUTIN
hydroxyurea	HYDREA
ibuprofen	MOTRIN, RUFEN
indomethacin	INDOCIN
isoxsuprine	VASODILAN
kanamycin	KANTREX
levopropoxyphene	NOVRAD
lomustine	CeeNU
loperamide	IMODIUM
mafenide	SULFAMYLON
mechlorethamine	MUSTARGEN
medroxyprogesterone	AMEN
megestrol	MEGACE
melphalan	ALKERAN
meperidine	DEMEROL
mercaptopurine	PURINETHOL
methicillin	STAPHCILLIN
methotrexate	MEXATE
methyclothiazide	AQUATENSEN, ENDURON
methyldopa	ALDOMET
methylergonovine	METHERGINE
metolazone	DIULO, ZAROXOLYN
metoprolol	LOPRESSOR

(continued)

GLOSSARY OF GENERIC AND TRADE NAMES (continued)

metronidazole	FLAGYL
mezlocillin	MEZLIN
miconazole	MONISTAT
moxalactam	MOXAM
nadolol	CORGARD
nafcillin	NAFCIL, UNIPEN
naproxen	ANAPROX, NAPROSYN
neomycin	MYCIFRADIN, NEOBIOTIC, MYCIQUENT
nitrazepam	MOGADON
noscapine	ISOFIL
nystatin	MYCOSTATIN, NILSTAT, O-V STATIN
oxacillin	PROSTAPHLIN
oxazepam	SERAX
oxycodone	PERCODAN
oxymorphone	NUMORPHAN
oxytocin	PITOCIN, SYNTOCINON
penicillin G procaine	CRYSTICILLIN, DURACILLIN, others
penicillin V potassium	COMPOCILLIN-V K, PEN-VEE K, others
pentazocine	TALWIN
pentobarbital	NEMBUTAL
phenobarbital	LUMINAL
phenoxybenzamine	DIBENZYLINE
phentolamine	REGITINE
phenylbutazone	AZOLID, BUTAZOLIDIN
piperacillin	PIPRACIL
polythiazide	RENESE
prazosin	MINIPRESS
probenecid	BENEMID
propranolol	INDERAL
propoxyphene	DARVON, SK-65
pyrimethamine	DARAPRIM
quinethazone	HYDROMOX
reserpine	SERPASIL

(continued)

GLOSSARY OF GENERIC AND TRADE NAMES (continued)

ritodrine	YUTOPAR
secobarbital	SECONAL
silver sulfadiazine	SILVADENE
sodium nitroprusside	NIPRIDE, NITROPRESS
spironolactone	ALDACTONE
sulfacetamide	SULTRIN
sulfacytine	RENOQUID
sulfadiazine	SULADYNE
sulfamethizole	MICROSUL, THIOSULFIL
sulfamethoxazole (combination with trimethoprim)	BACTRIM, SEPTRA
sulfasalazine	AZULFIDINE
sulfisoxazole	GANTRISIN
sulindac	CLINORIL
tamoxifen	NOLVADEX
terbutaline	BRETHINE, BRICANYL
testosterone	ORETON, others
thiopental	PENTOTHAL
ticarcillin	TICAR
tobramycin	NEBCIN
tolmetin	TOLECTIN
triamterene	DYRENIUM
trichlormethiazide	METAHYDRIN, NAQUA
trimethoprim	PROLOPRIM, TRIMPEX
vinblastine	VELBAN
vincristine	ONCOVIN
vindesine	ELDISINE

Index